Healthy Living:

A Comprehensive Weight Loss Guide

By Evelyn Inkwell

To all the people out there who are still trying

INTRODUCTION

In a world inundated with fad diets, quick fixes, and miracle supplements promising overnight transformations, the pursuit of weight loss can feel like an endless maze of confusion and disappointment. Yet, buried beneath the noise of sensationalized headlines and glossy magazine covers lies a fundamental truth: sustainable weight loss is not about drastic measures or temporary solutions. It's about adopting a balanced, holistic approach that nurtures both body and mind.

Welcome to "Healthy Living: A Comprehensive Weight Loss Guide." In the pages that follow, we embark on a journey that transcends the superficial allure of crash diets and fleeting trends. Instead, we delve deep into the core principles of long-term weight management, offering you the tools, knowledge, and support needed to transform your relationship with food, exercise, and self.

Before we embark on this transformative journey together, it's essential to acknowledge the underlying motivations that often drive our desire for weight loss. While the pursuit of a healthier body is undoubtedly commendable, it's crucial to approach this journey with a mindset rooted in self-love and acceptance. We are not embarking on this journey to conform to societal standards of beauty or to attain an unattainable ideal. Rather, we are committing to prioritize our health and well-being, honoring the magnificent vessel that carries us through life.

At the heart of sustainable weight loss lies the understanding that it is not a destination but a lifelong journey. It's about making gradual, sustainable changes that align with our individual needs, preferences, and goals. Whether you're looking to shed excess pounds, improve your overall health, or simply feel more confident in your skin, the principles outlined in this book are designed to empower you to reclaim control over your body and your life.

Throughout these pages, we will explore the science behind weight loss, debunking common myths and misconceptions along the way. From understanding the role of calories and metabolism to mastering the art of mindful eating, each chapter is packed with evidence-based strategies and practical tips to help you navigate the complexities of weight management with confidence and clarity.

But this journey is about more than just numbers on a scale or inches lost. It's about embracing a holistic approach to health that encompasses not only the physical but also the mental and emotional aspects of well-being. We will delve into the psychological barriers that often sabotage our efforts, offering insights and techniques to overcome self-doubt, emotional eating, and negative self-talk.

Furthermore, we will explore the importance of self-care, stress management, and sleep hygiene in supporting our weight loss journey. By prioritizing our physical and mental health, we lay the foundation for sustainable success, fostering resilience and empowerment every step of the way.

As we embark on this journey together, I invite you to approach it with an open mind and a compassionate heart. Remember that transformation is not always linear, and setbacks are merely opportunities for growth and learning. By cultivating patience, perseverance, and self-compassion, you will discover the power within you to create lasting change and live your healthiest, happiest life.

So, let us embark on this journey of transformation together, one step at a time, one choice at a time. Together, we will unlock the untapped potential within you, guiding you towards a future filled with vitality, confidence, and boundless possibilities. Are you ready to transform your body and your life? Let's begin.

CHAPTER 1: THE IMPORTANCE OF A HEALTHY WEIGHT AND ITS IMPACT ON OVERALL WELL-BEING

In today's fast-paced world, it's easy to overlook the importance of maintaining a healthy weight amidst the chaos of daily life. However, the significance of achieving and maintaining a healthy weight cannot be overstated, as it plays a pivotal role in shaping our overall well-being, both physically and mentally. In this chapter, we will explore the profound impact that weight has on our health, longevity, and quality of life, and delve into the multifaceted benefits of achieving a balanced weight.

At its core, achieving a healthy weight is not merely about conforming to societal standards of beauty or attaining a certain clothing size. Instead, it's about optimizing our physical health and reducing our risk of developing chronic diseases that can significantly compromise our quality of life. Excess weight, particularly when concentrated around the abdomen, has been linked to a myriad of health issues, including heart disease, type 2 diabetes, stroke, and certain types of cancer. By shedding excess pounds and maintaining a healthy weight, we can significantly reduce our risk of developing these life-threatening conditions, thus enhancing our overall health and longevity.

Moreover, the benefits of achieving a healthy weight extend far beyond physical health, encompassing mental and emotional well-being as well. Research has consistently shown that individuals who maintain a healthy weight are more likely to experience improved mood, higher self-esteem, and enhanced overall quality of life. Conversely, those who struggle with obesity or overweight often grapple with feelings of shame, guilt, and low self-worth, which can perpetuate a vicious cycle of emotional eating and further exacerbate weight-related issues.

Furthermore, achieving a healthy weight can have profound implications for our day-to-day functioning and vitality. Excess weight can place undue strain on our joints, leading to chronic pain and mobility issues that can significantly impair our ability to engage in physical activity and enjoy life to the fullest. By shedding excess pounds and alleviating this burden on our bodies, we can experience newfound energy, vitality, and resilience, enabling us to embrace life's adventures with renewed vigor and enthusiasm.

In addition to the physical and emotional benefits of achieving a healthy weight, there are also significant financial implications to consider. The economic burden of obesity and overweight is staggering, with healthcare costs associated with weight-related conditions reaching astronomical levels each year. By taking proactive steps to achieve and maintain a healthy weight, individuals can potentially mitigate these healthcare costs, freeing up financial resources for other priorities and investments in their health and well-being.

Furthermore, achieving a healthy weight is not merely a personal endeavor but also a collective responsibility that impacts society as a whole. The ripple effects of obesity extend far beyond individual health outcomes, encompassing broader societal issues such as healthcare disparities, environmental sustainability, and economic productivity. By promoting policies and initiatives that support healthy eating, active living, and equitable access to resources, we can create a culture of health and well-being that benefits everyone, regardless of socioeconomic status or background.

In conclusion, the importance of achieving and maintaining a healthy weight cannot be overstated. From reducing our risk of chronic diseases to enhancing our mental and emotional well-being, the benefits of achieving a balanced weight are profound and far-reaching. By prioritizing our health and taking proactive steps to nurture our bodies, we not only enhance our own well-being but also contribute to a healthier, happier society for generations to come.

CHAPTER 2: UNDERSTANDING WEIGHT LOSS

In our quest for weight loss, it's crucial to understand the underlying scientific principles that govern our bodies' response to food, energy expenditure, and metabolism. By gaining insight into the intricate mechanisms at play, we can make informed decisions and adopt effective strategies for achieving sustainable results. In this chapter, we will delve deep into the science behind weight loss, exploring the roles of calories, metabolism, genetics, and body composition in shaping our bodies and influencing our weight.

Calories: The Currency of Energy

At the heart of weight management lies a fundamental concept: calories, the currency of energy that powers our bodies' myriad functions. Calories serve as the basic unit of measurement for the energy content of foods, determining the balance between energy intake and expenditure. Put simply, weight loss occurs when we consume fewer calories than we expend, creating a caloric deficit that prompts our bodies to utilize stored energy reserves, primarily in the form of fat, to meet its energy needs. Conversely, weight gain ensues when we consume more calories than we burn, leading to the accumulation of excess energy in the form of fat tissue.

Understanding the role of calories in weight management is paramount for achieving and sustaining a healthy weight. While it's true that not all calories are created equal – with variations in the quality of nutrients and macronutrient composition influencing overall health – the fundamental principle of energy balance remains steadfast. To achieve weight loss, it's imperative to establish a sustainable caloric deficit through a combination of dietary adjustments and increased physical activity.

Dietary modifications play a central role in creating a caloric deficit. This involves making mindful choices about the types and quantities of foods we consume, prioritizing nutrient-dense options while minimizing empty calories from processed foods, sugary beverages, and unhealthy fats. By focusing on whole, unprocessed foods rich in fiber, vitamins, and minerals, we can optimize satiety and nutritional intake, supporting overall health and weight management goals.

In addition to dietary modifications, increasing physical activity is another essential component of achieving a caloric deficit and promoting weight loss. Exercise not only burns calories directly but also enhances metabolic rate and contributes to lean muscle mass development, both of which can facilitate weight loss and improve body composition. Incorporating a combination of cardiovascular exercise, strength training, and flexibility exercises into our routine can maximize calorie expenditure and promote sustainable weight loss over time.

Furthermore, adopting mindful eating practices can help us tune into our body's hunger and satiety cues, fostering a more intuitive approach to food consumption and promoting healthier eating habits in the long term. By practicing mindful eating, we can cultivate a deeper awareness of our dietary choices, savor the sensory experience of eating, and foster a more positive relationship with food.

In conclusion, calories serve as the cornerstone of weight management, dictating the delicate balance between energy intake and expenditure. By creating a sustainable caloric deficit through dietary modifications, increased physical activity, and mindful eating practices, we can achieve and maintain a healthy weight while supporting overall health and well-being. Remember, achieving lasting results requires patience, consistency, and a holistic approach that prioritizes both physical and mental well-being.

Metabolism: The Body's Engine

Metabolism, often described as the body's internal engine, orchestrates a complex symphony of biochemical processes that transform food into the energy necessary to fuel our daily activities. This intricate network of metabolic pathways plays a central role in determining our bodies' energy needs and exerting a profound influence on our weight management journey.

At the core of metabolism lies the concept of basal metabolic rate (BMR), also known as resting metabolic rate (RMR). BMR represents the minimum number of calories required by our bodies to sustain essential physiological functions while at rest, such as breathing, circulating blood, and maintaining body temperature. This baseline level of energy expenditure varies from person to person and is influenced by a variety of factors, including age, gender, body composition, and genetics.

One critical determinant of BMR is lean muscle mass. Muscle tissue is metabolically active, meaning it requires more energy to maintain than fat tissue. Therefore, individuals with a higher proportion of lean muscle mass tend to have a higher BMR, as their bodies expend more calories at rest to support muscle function and repair. This underscores the importance of incorporating strength training exercises into our fitness routine to preserve and build lean muscle mass, thereby enhancing metabolic rate and supporting weight management efforts.

In addition to BMR, two other components contribute to total energy expenditure: physical activity and the thermic effect of food (TEF). Physical activity encompasses both structured exercise, such as jogging or weightlifting, and non-exercise activity thermogenesis (NEAT), which encompasses the energy expended during daily activities such as fidgeting, walking, and standing. By engaging in regular physical activity, we not only burn calories directly but also stimulate metabolic adaptations that can further enhance energy expenditure and promote weight loss.

Similarly, the thermic effect of food refers to the energy expended during the process of digestion, absorption, and metabolism of food. Different macronutrients have varying thermic effects, with protein requiring more energy to digest and metabolize compared to carbohydrates or fats. By incorporating lean protein sources into our meals, such as poultry, fish, tofu, or legumes, we can maximize the thermic effect of food and support our weight loss efforts.

By understanding the interplay between these components of metabolism – BMR, physical activity, and TEF – we can optimize our energy balance and create an environment conducive to weight loss. By incorporating a combination of dietary modifications, increased physical activity, and muscle-building exercises into our lifestyle, we can support metabolic health, enhance energy expenditure, and achieve sustainable weight loss results.

In conclusion, metabolism serves as a cornerstone of weight management, dictating our bodies' energy needs and influencing our ability to achieve and maintain a healthy weight. By understanding the factors that influence metabolism – such as BMR, physical activity, and the thermic effect of food – we can implement targeted strategies to optimize energy balance and support our weight loss journey. Remember, achieving lasting results requires a holistic approach that prioritizes both diet and exercise, along with consistency, patience, and a commitment to long-term lifestyle changes.

Genetics: Unraveling the Genetic Code

While lifestyle choices like diet and exercise undoubtedly wield considerable influence over weight management, genetics stands as a formidable force, shaping our predisposition to obesity and influencing how our bodies respond to weight loss interventions. Through extensive research, scientists have uncovered a plethora of genetic variants linked to an elevated risk of obesity. These variants often impact key aspects of metabolism and appetite regulation, dictating how efficiently our bodies process energy and manage hunger cues.

Among the genetic factors implicated in obesity risk are those involved in appetite regulation. Variants in genes related to appetite hormones such as leptin and ghrelin can alter how our bodies signal hunger and satiety, potentially leading to overeating and weight gain. Additionally, genetic variations affecting energy expenditure, such as those influencing thyroid function or mitochondrial efficiency, can influence our bodies' ability to burn calories and regulate weight. Furthermore, alterations in genes involved in fat metabolism can impact how efficiently our bodies store or utilize fat, contributing to weight gain and obesity risk.

Despite the significant impact of genetics on weight management, it's crucial to recognize that our genetic makeup is not our destiny. While we may inherit certain predispositions towards weight gain or obesity, our lifestyle choices and environmental factors play a pivotal role in shaping our bodies and influencing our health outcomes. By adopting healthy habits and making sustainable lifestyle changes, we can mitigate genetic risk factors and optimize our overall well-being.

One key strategy for overcoming genetic predispositions to obesity is to prioritize a balanced diet rich in nutrient-dense foods. By focusing on whole, unprocessed foods and incorporating plenty of fruits, vegetables, lean proteins, and healthy fats into our meals, we can support metabolic health and promote weight management. Additionally, paying attention to portion sizes and practicing mindful eating can help regulate calorie intake and prevent overeating, regardless of genetic predispositions.

Regular physical activity also plays a crucial role in mitigating genetic risk factors for obesity. Exercise not only burns calories and promotes weight loss but also triggers beneficial metabolic adaptations that can counteract genetic predispositions towards weight gain. By engaging in a combination of aerobic exercise, strength training, and flexibility exercises, we can support metabolic health, build lean muscle mass, and enhance overall well-being.

Furthermore, adopting stress management techniques and prioritizing adequate sleep can help mitigate the impact of genetic factors on weight management. Chronic stress and sleep deprivation can disrupt hormonal balance and increase appetite, potentially exacerbating genetic predispositions towards obesity. By incorporating stress-reducing activities such as meditation, yoga, or deep breathing exercises into our daily routine and prioritizing restful sleep, we can support metabolic health and optimize our weight management efforts.

In conclusion, while genetics undoubtedly plays a significant role in shaping our predisposition to obesity, it is not the sole determinant of our weight destiny. By adopting healthy habits, making sustainable lifestyle changes, and prioritizing factors within our control such as diet, exercise, stress management, and sleep, we can mitigate genetic risk factors and optimize our overall well-being. With dedication, perseverance, and a holistic approach to health, we can overcome genetic predispositions and achieve lasting success in weight management.

Body Composition: Beyond the Scale

When embarking on a journey of weight management, it's imperative to recognize that the scale tells only a fraction of the story. Beyond mere weight, understanding our body composition – the intricate interplay of fat, muscle, bone, and other tissues – is essential for achieving holistic health and well-being. While conventional wisdom often equates weight loss with fat loss, the reality is far more nuanced, with changes in body composition influenced by a multitude of factors, including diet, exercise, and hormonal fluctuations.

One crucial aspect of body composition management is the preservation of lean muscle mass during weight loss. Unlike fat, which serves primarily as a storage depot for excess energy, muscle tissue is metabolically active, playing a vital role in supporting metabolic health and overall well-being. Resistance training emerges as a powerful tool for preserving lean muscle mass while promoting fat loss. Unlike traditional cardiovascular exercises, which primarily target calorie expenditure, resistance training elicits muscle growth and metabolic adaptations that can enhance overall metabolic rate and improve body composition.

Engaging in resistance training stimulates muscle protein synthesis, the process by which new muscle tissue is created, leading to increases in muscle mass and strength. Additionally, resistance exercises promote the activation of fast-twitch muscle fibers, which are particularly adept at burning calories and supporting fat loss. By incorporating a variety of resistance exercises – such as weightlifting, bodyweight exercises, and resistance bands – into our fitness routine, we can stimulate muscle growth, enhance metabolic function, and achieve a more sculpted and toned physique.

Moreover, resistance training triggers beneficial metabolic adaptations that extend beyond the gym, influencing our bodies' energy expenditure and fat-burning capabilities throughout the day. By increasing muscle mass, resistance exercises elevate basal metabolic rate (BMR), the number of calories our bodies expend at rest, thereby facilitating fat loss and supporting weight management efforts. Additionally, resistance training enhances insulin sensitivity, the ability of our cells to respond to insulin and regulate blood sugar levels, which can reduce the risk of obesity and metabolic disorders.

Incorporating a balanced exercise regimen that includes both cardiovascular exercise and resistance training is key to achieving optimal body composition and promoting overall health and well-being. Cardiovascular exercise, such as running, cycling, or swimming, helps burn calories, improve cardiovascular health, and enhance endurance. However, to maximize fat loss and preserve lean muscle mass, it's essential to complement cardiovascular exercise with regular resistance training sessions.

Furthermore, flexibility exercises, such as yoga or stretching, can help improve joint mobility, reduce the risk of injury, and enhance overall physical performance. By integrating a diverse array of exercise modalities into our routine – including cardiovascular exercise, resistance training, and flexibility exercises – we can achieve a comprehensive approach to weight management that prioritizes both fat loss and muscle preservation.

In conclusion, when it comes to weight management, focusing solely on the number on the scale overlooks the importance of body composition. By incorporating resistance training into our fitness routine, we can preserve lean muscle mass, promote fat loss, and support metabolic health. By embracing a holistic approach that encompasses cardiovascular exercise, resistance training, and flexibility exercises, we can achieve optimal body composition, enhance overall well-being, and unlock our full potential for health and vitality.

Weight loss is a multifaceted process governed by a complex interplay of factors, including calories, metabolism, genetics, and body composition. By understanding the underlying science behind weight loss, we can make informed decisions and adopt effective strategies for achieving sustainable results. By creating a caloric deficit through dietary modifications and increased physical activity, optimizing metabolic rate through lifestyle interventions, and addressing genetic and body composition factors, we can embark on a journey towards improved health and well-being. Remember, there is no one-size-fits-all approach to weight loss, and it's essential to tailor our approach to our individual needs, preferences, and goals. With dedication, perseverance, and a solid understanding of the science behind weight loss, we can achieve lasting success and unlock our full potential for health and vitality.

CHAPTER 3: SETTING REALISTIC GOALS

Setting achievable weight loss goals is a crucial step in embarking on a successful journey towards a healthier lifestyle. However, it's essential to approach goal-setting with a realistic mindset and a clear understanding of what it takes to achieve sustainable results. In this chapter, we will explore the principles of effective goal-setting, provide practical strategies for setting achievable weight loss goals, and offer guidance on how to stay motivated and focused throughout the process.

The Importance of Setting Realistic Goals

Setting realistic goals is paramount for long-term success in weight loss. Unrealistic or overly ambitious goals can lead to frustration, disappointment, and ultimately, abandonment of our efforts. Instead, it's essential to set goals that are both challenging yet attainable, taking into account our individual circumstances, lifestyle, and preferences.

When setting weight loss goals, it's helpful to consider both short-term and long-term objectives. Short-term goals provide a roadmap for immediate progress and help us stay motivated by celebrating small victories along the way. Long-term goals, on the other hand, provide a broader vision for our journey and serve as a source of inspiration and direction.

SMART Goal Setting

A widely used framework for setting achievable goals is the SMART criteria, which stands for Specific, Measurable, Achievable, Relevant, and Time-bound. By applying these principles to our weight loss goals, we can ensure clarity, accountability, and effectiveness in our approach.

- **Specific**: Clearly define what you want to achieve. Instead of a vague goal like "lose weight," specify the amount of weight you aim to lose and the timeframe in which you plan to achieve it.

- **Measurable**: Establish concrete criteria for tracking your progress. This could involve tracking your weight on a weekly basis, measuring inches lost, or monitoring changes in body composition using tools like body fat calipers or a DEXA scan.

- **Achievable**: Set goals that are within your reach. Consider factors such as your current weight, health status, lifestyle, and available resources when determining what is achievable for you.

- **Relevant**: Ensure that your goals align with your values, priorities, and overall well-being. Ask yourself why this goal is important to you and how achieving it will enhance your life.

- **Time-bound**: Establish a deadline or timeframe for achieving your goals. This creates a sense of urgency and helps keep you focused and motivated.

Breaking Down Goals into Actionable Steps

Once you've established your overarching weight loss goals, break them down into smaller, actionable steps. This makes your goals more manageable and helps prevent overwhelm. For example, if your long-term goal is to lose 50 pounds in six months, break it down into monthly or weekly targets, such as losing 2 pounds per week or 8 pounds per month.

Each actionable step should be specific, measurable, and achievable, with a clear plan of action for implementation. For instance, if one of your goals is to incorporate more physical activity into your daily routine, you might start by scheduling regular workouts, joining a fitness class, or setting aside time for brisk walks during your lunch break.

Tracking Progress and Adjusting Goals

Regularly monitoring your progress is essential for staying on track and making adjustments as needed. Keep track of your weight, measurements, exercise habits, dietary choices, and other relevant metrics to gauge your progress towards your goals. Use a journal, smartphone app, or spreadsheet to record your daily activities and track your results over time.

Be flexible and willing to adjust your goals as you progress. If you find that you're consistently falling short of your targets, reassess your approach and consider making modifications to your goals or action plan. Conversely, if you're exceeding your expectations, challenge yourself to set new, more ambitious goals that push you out of your comfort zone.

Celebrating Achievements and Staying Motivated

Celebrate your achievements along the way, no matter how small. Acknowledge your progress, reward yourself for reaching milestones, and celebrate your successes with friends, family, or support groups. Positive reinforcement can boost motivation and reinforce healthy habits, making it easier to stay committed to your goals over the long term.

Additionally, find sources of inspiration and motivation that resonate with you. Whether it's reading success stories, following fitness influencers on social media, or visualizing your goals through vision boards or affirmations, surround yourself with positivity and encouragement that fuel your determination and keep you focused on your objectives.

Setting achievable weight loss goals is a critical first step in embarking on a journey towards a healthier, happier life. By applying the principles of SMART goal setting, breaking down goals into actionable steps, tracking progress, and staying motivated, you can set yourself up for success and achieve sustainable results. Remember, the journey towards better health is not always linear, and setbacks are a natural part of the process. Be patient, stay persistent, and trust in your ability to overcome obstacles and reach your goals. With dedication, perseverance, and a clear vision for your future, you can transform your body and your life.

However, the effectiveness of goal-setting lies not only in establishing objectives but also in the differentiation between short-term and long-term goals. In this chapter, we will delve into the significance of setting both short-term and long-term goals, exploring how each contributes to the success of our journey towards a healthier lifestyle.

Understanding Short-Term Goals

Short-term goals provide the stepping stones that propel us forward on our path to long-term success. These goals typically cover a timeframe of days, weeks, or months and focus on immediate progress and tangible achievements. Short-term goals serve several essential functions in the weight loss journey:

1. Motivation and Momentum:

Short-term goals act as catalysts for motivation, providing us with regular opportunities to experience the satisfaction of achievement. By setting achievable targets within a relatively short timeframe, we maintain a sense of momentum and progress, which fuels our motivation to continue working towards our long-term objectives.

2. Building Habits:

Short-term goals serve as building blocks for establishing healthy habits. By breaking down our long-term aspirations into smaller, actionable steps, we create opportunities to practice and reinforce positive behaviors consistently. Whether it's committing to regular exercise, adopting healthier eating habits, or prioritizing self-care, short-term goals provide the structure and accountability needed to cultivate lasting lifestyle changes.

3. Course Correction:

Short-term goals allow for flexibility and adaptability in our approach. If we encounter obstacles or setbacks along the way, short-term goals enable us to reassess our strategies, make necessary adjustments, and course-correct as needed. This iterative process of trial and error empowers us to learn from our experiences, refine our methods, and ultimately, progress towards our long-term goals more effectively.

Embracing the Power of Long-Term Goals

While short-term goals provide the immediate focus and momentum needed to propel us forward, long-term goals offer a broader vision and sense of purpose that guides our journey over time. Long-term goals typically span months, years, or even decades and reflect our overarching aspirations and aspirations for the future. Here's why long-term goals are essential:

1. Providing Direction and Clarity:
Long-term goals serve as beacons that guide our actions and decisions, providing us with a clear sense of direction and purpose. By articulating our ultimate objectives — whether it's achieving a specific weight, completing a marathon, or reclaiming our overall health — long-term goals help us stay focused and committed, even in the face of challenges or distractions.

2. Sustaining Motivation and Resilience:
Long-term goals inspire us to persevere and overcome obstacles, even when the journey becomes difficult or arduous. By connecting our daily efforts to our broader aspirations for the future, long-term goals imbue our actions with meaning and significance, sustaining our motivation and resilience throughout the ups and downs of the weight loss journey.

3. Fostering Accountability and Commitment:
Long-term goals create a sense of accountability and commitment to ourselves, our health, and our well-being. By publicly declaring our long-term intentions and aspirations, whether to friends, family, or ourselves, we establish a sense of ownership and responsibility for our actions, reinforcing our commitment to achieving our goals and maintaining our progress over time.

Achieving Balance and Integration
While short-term and long-term goals serve distinct purposes in our weight loss journey, they are not mutually exclusive. Instead, they complement and reinforce each other, forming a cohesive framework that guides our actions and shapes our outcomes. Achieving balance and integration between short-term and long-term goals requires a holistic approach that considers both immediate needs and future aspirations:

1. Aligning Short-Term Goals with Long-Term Objectives:
To maximize the effectiveness of short-term goals, ensure that they are aligned with your long-term aspirations and priorities. Each short-term goal should contribute directly to the achievement of your overarching long-term goals, serving as incremental steps towards your desired outcome.

2. Periodic Review and Reflection:
Regularly review and reflect on your progress towards both your short-term and long-term goals. Celebrate your achievements, identify areas for improvement, and adjust your goals and strategies as needed to stay on track and maintain momentum towards your ultimate objectives.

3. Flexibility and Adaptability:
Be open to adapting your goals and strategies in response to changing circumstances, priorities, or preferences. While long-term goals provide a guiding vision, it's essential to remain flexible and responsive to new opportunities, challenges, and insights that may arise along the way.

In conclusion, setting both short-term and long-term goals is essential for achieving success in our weight loss journey. Short-term goals provide the immediate focus, motivation, and momentum needed to propel us forward, while long-term goals offer a broader vision and sense of purpose that guides our actions and sustains our commitment over time. By striking a balance between short-term progress and long-term aspirations, we can create a holistic framework that empowers us to achieve lasting success in our pursuit of a healthier, happier life. Remember, the journey towards better health is not a sprint but a marathon, and by setting achievable goals and staying focused on our long-term vision, we can overcome obstacles, persevere through challenges, and ultimately, transform our lives for the better.

CHAPTER 4: OVERCOMING MENTAL BARRIERS

Embarking on a journey towards weight loss often involves more than just physical challenges; it requires navigating a complex landscape of mental and emotional obstacles that can hinder our progress and undermine our efforts. In this chapter, we will explore some of the most common mental obstacles to weight loss, including negative self-talk and emotional eating, and provide strategies for overcoming them to achieve lasting success.

Negative Self-Talk: The Inner Critic

One of the most pervasive mental obstacles to weight loss is negative self-talk – the inner dialogue of self-criticism, doubt, and self-limiting beliefs that can erode our confidence and motivation. Negative self-talk often takes the form of harsh judgments, comparisons to others, and distorted perceptions of our bodies and abilities. Left unchecked, it can sabotage our efforts and undermine our self-esteem, making it difficult to stay committed to our weight loss goals.

Recognizing Negative Self-Talk:

Negative self-talk can be insidious, creeping into our minds and eroding our confidence without us even realizing it. The first crucial step in combating this destructive pattern is to bring it into the light of awareness. By recognizing negative self-talk for what it is – a harmful cycle of thought that undermines our well-being and hinders our success – we can begin to dismantle its power over us.

To recognize negative self-talk, it's essential to tune into the language and tone of our inner dialogue. Notice any recurring themes of self-criticism, doubt, or defeatism that arise throughout your day. Are there certain phrases or beliefs that frequently surface when you face challenges or setbacks? Do you find yourself engaging in harsh self-judgment or comparing yourself unfavorably to others? By paying attention to these patterns, you can start to identify the ways in which negative self-talk manifests in your thoughts and perceptions.

Once you've identified negative self-talk, the next step is to challenge and reframe it in more constructive and empowering ways. This involves questioning the validity of the negative thoughts and beliefs that arise and replacing them with more positive and affirming alternatives. For example, if you catch yourself thinking, "I'll never be good enough," challenge this belief by asking yourself, "Is this thought based on facts or my own insecurities?" Then, replace it with a more empowering affirmation, such as, "I am capable and deserving of success."

Another effective strategy for reframing negative self-talk is to practice self-compassion. Treat yourself with the same kindness, understanding, and support you would offer to a friend in a similar situation. Instead of berating yourself for perceived shortcomings or failures, offer yourself words of encouragement and reassurance. Remind yourself that it's natural to face challenges and setbacks along the way, and that your worth is not determined by your achievements or perceived flaws.

In addition to challenging and reframing negative self-talk, it's essential to cultivate a supportive inner dialogue that fosters self-confidence and resilience. This involves cultivating a sense of self-worth and self-acceptance, regardless of external validation or approval. Recognize and celebrate your strengths, accomplishments, and progress, no matter how small. Focus on your unique qualities and talents, and embrace yourself with love and appreciation.

Practicing gratitude can also be a powerful antidote to negative self-talk. Take time each day to reflect on the things you're grateful for, whether it's the support of loved ones, the beauty of nature, or the simple pleasures of life. Cultivating an attitude of gratitude can shift your focus away from negativity and scarcity towards positivity and abundance, fostering a more resilient mindset in the face of challenges.

In conclusion, overcoming negative self-talk requires self-awareness, self-compassion, and a commitment to challenging and reframing unhelpful thought patterns. By recognizing negative self-talk for what it is, challenging its validity, and replacing it with more constructive alternatives, we can break free from its grip and cultivate a more positive and empowering inner dialogue. Remember that change takes time and effort, so be patient and gentle with yourself as you embark on this journey of self-discovery and growth. With practice and perseverance, you can transform your inner narrative and unlock your full potential for success and well-being.

Cultivating Self-Compassion:
One of the most potent antidotes to negative self-talk is the practice of self-compassion. At its core, self-compassion entails treating oneself with the same kindness, understanding, and acceptance that we would extend to a cherished friend or loved one. Especially in moments of struggle or setback, when our inner critic is loudest, self-compassion offers a gentle and supportive alternative to self-judgment and criticism.

Instead of succumbing to the impulse to berate ourselves for perceived failures or shortcomings, self-compassion encourages us to respond with empathy and understanding. Imagine how you would comfort and support a dear friend who was facing a similar challenge. You would likely offer words of encouragement, reassurance, and compassion, reminding them that setbacks are a natural part of the journey and that their worth is not defined by their mistakes or struggles. By extending this same level of compassion to ourselves, we can cultivate a more nurturing and supportive inner dialogue.

It's important to remember that weight loss is not a linear path, but rather a journey filled with ups and downs, twists and turns. Setbacks are an inevitable part of the process, and they do not diminish our worth or value as individuals. Approach yourself with patience, kindness, and encouragement, knowing that you are worthy of love and acceptance regardless of your weight or appearance. By embracing self-compassion, we can create a space of safety and acceptance within ourselves, allowing us to navigate the challenges of weight loss with greater resilience and self-assurance.

In moments of struggle or self-doubt, self-compassion serves as a powerful anchor, grounding us in a sense of worthiness and belonging. Rather than striving for perfection or punishing ourselves for perceived failures, self-compassion encourages us to embrace our humanity – flaws, mistakes, and all – with open-hearted acceptance and kindness. By offering ourselves the same level of compassion and support that we would offer to a dear friend, we can foster a deeper sense of self-acceptance and resilience, enabling us to navigate the challenges of weight loss with greater grace and ease.

Practicing self-compassion does not mean ignoring or minimizing the difficulties we face. Instead, it involves acknowledging our struggles with honesty and gentleness, while also recognizing our inherent worth and dignity as human beings. Self-compassion allows us to hold ourselves accountable for our actions and choices without resorting to harsh self-judgment or criticism. It invites us to approach ourselves with kindness and understanding, even in moments of failure or setback, knowing that we are doing the best we can with the resources and knowledge we have available to us.

In conclusion, self-compassion is a powerful antidote to negative self-talk, offering a gentle and supportive alternative to self-criticism and judgment. By treating ourselves with kindness, understanding, and acceptance, especially in moments of struggle or setback, we can cultivate a deeper sense of self-worth and resilience. Remember that weight loss is a journey, and setbacks are a natural part of the process. Approach yourself with patience, kindness, and encouragement, knowing that you are worthy of love and acceptance regardless of your weight or appearance.

Reframing Limiting Beliefs:
Challenging and reframing limiting beliefs is a pivotal step in combating negative self-talk and cultivating a mindset of self-confidence and resilience. Limiting beliefs are deeply ingrained assumptions or perceptions about ourselves and our abilities that hold us back from reaching our full potential. They often manifest as self-defeating statements such as "I'll never be able to lose weight" or "I'm not capable of sticking to a healthy lifestyle." By questioning the validity of these beliefs and replacing them with more empowering affirmations, we can shift our mindset and pave the way for positive change.

The first step in challenging limiting beliefs is to question their accuracy and validity. Ask yourself, "Is this belief based on facts or assumptions?" Often, limiting beliefs are rooted in past experiences, societal norms, or unfounded fears rather than objective reality. By examining the evidence and challenging the logic behind these beliefs, we can begin to dismantle their hold on our thinking.

Once we've identified and questioned our limiting beliefs, the next step is to replace them with more empowering and realistic affirmations. Instead of saying, "I'll never be able to lose weight," reframe it as "I am capable of making positive changes in my life." This shift in perspective acknowledges our potential for growth and transformation, empowering us to take proactive steps towards achieving our goals.

Similarly, instead of saying, "I'm not capable of sticking to a healthy lifestyle," replace it with "Every small step I take brings me closer to my goals." This affirmation recognizes the importance of progress over perfection and celebrates the incremental changes we make towards living a healthier life. By focusing on the small victories and milestones along the way, we can stay motivated and build momentum towards our larger goals.

In addition to reframing limiting beliefs with affirmations, it's essential to consciously choose to focus on our strengths, successes, and potential for growth. Take inventory of your accomplishments, skills, and positive attributes, and remind yourself of them regularly. By highlighting our strengths and successes, we can bolster our self-confidence and resilience, making it easier to overcome challenges and setbacks along the way.

Furthermore, cultivate a growth mindset – the belief that our abilities and intelligence can be developed through dedication and effort. Embrace challenges as opportunities for learning and growth, rather than viewing them as threats to our self-worth or competence. By adopting a growth mindset, we can embrace the journey of self-improvement with enthusiasm and optimism, knowing that every obstacle we encounter is an opportunity to become stronger and more resilient.

In conclusion, challenging and reframing limiting beliefs is a powerful tool for overcoming negative self-talk and cultivating a mindset of self-confidence and resilience. By questioning the validity of our beliefs, replacing them with empowering affirmations, and focusing on our strengths and potential for growth, we can shift our mindset and pave the way for positive change. Remember that change takes time and effort, so be patient and persistent in your journey towards self-improvement. With dedication and a commitment to self-discovery, you can break free from the shackles of limiting beliefs and unleash your full potential for success and fulfillment.

Emotional Eating: Navigating the Comfort Zone

Another common mental obstacle to weight loss is emotional eating – the tendency to turn to food for comfort, stress relief, or distraction from unpleasant emotions. Emotional eating often involves consuming large quantities of high-calorie, comfort foods in response to feelings of boredom, loneliness, anxiety, or sadness, leading to guilt, shame, and further emotional distress.

Mindful Awareness:

Addressing emotional eating begins with cultivating mindful awareness of our eating habits and emotional triggers. This involves paying close attention to the thoughts, feelings, and sensations that precede and accompany our eating episodes. By bringing conscious awareness to our eating behaviors, we can begin to unravel the complex relationship between our emotions and our desire to eat.

The first step in cultivating mindful awareness is to become attuned to the cues and signals our body sends us regarding hunger and fullness. Pay attention to physical sensations such as stomach grumbling, lightheadedness, or fatigue, which may indicate genuine hunger. Similarly, notice when you start to feel satisfied or full during a meal, and stop eating before you reach the point of discomfort.

In addition to physical cues, it's essential to tune into the thoughts and emotions that drive our eating behaviors. Notice any patterns or associations between specific emotions – such as stress, sadness, boredom, or loneliness – and your desire to eat. Do you find yourself reaching for food when you're feeling anxious or overwhelmed? Or perhaps you turn to snacks for comfort when you're feeling sad or lonely? By identifying these emotional triggers, we can begin to untangle the underlying reasons behind our urge to eat.

Once we've identified our emotional triggers, the next step is to explore alternative ways of coping with difficult emotions that don't involve food. This could involve practicing relaxation techniques such as deep breathing, meditation, or progressive muscle relaxation to help alleviate stress and anxiety. Engaging in activities that bring us joy and fulfillment, such as spending time with loved ones, pursuing hobbies or interests, or immersing ourselves in nature, can also provide a much-needed emotional boost without resorting to food.

Another effective strategy for addressing emotional eating is to cultivate a toolbox of healthy coping mechanisms that we can turn to when the urge to eat strikes. This could include journaling about our thoughts and feelings, talking to a trusted friend or therapist, or engaging in physical activity such as going for a walk or practicing yoga. By finding healthy ways to soothe and support ourselves during times of emotional distress, we can break free from the cycle of emotional eating and develop more adaptive coping strategies.

In addition to cultivating mindful awareness and exploring alternative coping mechanisms, it's essential to practice self-compassion and kindness towards ourselves as we navigate the challenges of emotional eating. Rather than judging or criticizing ourselves for succumbing to food cravings, offer ourselves the same level of understanding and support that we would offer to a friend in a similar situation. Remember that emotional eating is often a coping mechanism for dealing with difficult emotions, and it's okay to seek comfort and solace in food from time to time.

In conclusion, addressing emotional eating requires cultivating mindful awareness of our eating habits and emotional triggers, exploring alternative coping mechanisms, and practicing self-compassion and kindness towards ourselves. By bringing conscious awareness to our eating behaviors, identifying our emotional triggers, and finding healthy ways to cope with difficult emotions, we can break free from the cycle of emotional eating and cultivate a healthier relationship with food and our emotions. Remember that change takes time and effort, so be patient and persistent in your journey towards greater self-awareness and emotional well-being. With dedication and a commitment to self-care, you can overcome emotional eating and reclaim control over your eating habits and overall health.

Building Emotional Resilience:
Developing strategies for coping with emotional distress that don't involve food is essential for breaking free from the cycle of emotional eating and fostering a healthier relationship with food and emotions. Turning to food for comfort in times of stress, sadness, or boredom can quickly become a habit, but by exploring alternative coping mechanisms, we can learn to soothe and support ourselves in healthier, more adaptive ways.

One effective strategy for coping with emotional distress is to engage in activities that bring us joy and fulfillment. Spend time with loved ones, whether it's chatting with a friend, cuddling with a pet, or enjoying quality time with family members. Connecting with others can provide comfort and support, helping to alleviate feelings of loneliness or isolation.

Additionally, practicing relaxation techniques such as deep breathing, meditation, or progressive muscle relaxation can help to calm the mind and body during times of stress. Take a few moments each day to engage in these practices, focusing on your breath and allowing yourself to let go of tension and worry. By incorporating relaxation techniques into your daily routine, you can cultivate a sense of inner peace and resilience that can help you navigate difficult emotions more effectively.

Pursuing hobbies and interests that nourish your soul can also be an effective way to cope with emotional distress without turning to food. Whether it's painting, gardening, playing music, or immersing yourself in nature, engaging in activities that bring you joy and fulfillment can provide a much-needed escape from the pressures of daily life. By tapping into your passions and interests, you can create moments of joy and contentment that help to balance out the challenges and stresses of everyday living.

By building emotional resilience and expanding your repertoire of coping mechanisms, you can reduce reliance on food as a source of comfort and find healthier ways to manage your emotions. Remember that emotional eating is often a habit that develops over time, so breaking free from this pattern may take time and effort. Be patient with yourself as you explore alternative coping strategies and find what works best for you.

In conclusion, developing strategies for coping with emotional distress that don't involve food is essential for breaking free from the cycle of emotional eating and fostering a healthier relationship with food and emotions. By engaging in activities that bring you joy and fulfillment, practicing relaxation techniques, and pursuing hobbies and interests that nourish your soul, you can learn to soothe and support yourself in healthier, more adaptive ways. Remember that change takes time and effort, so be patient with yourself as you explore new coping strategies and find what works best for you. With dedication and perseverance, you can overcome emotional eating and cultivate a greater sense of emotional well-being and resilience.

Cultivating Self-Compassion:
Practicing self-compassion is a powerful tool for addressing the underlying emotional needs that drive emotional eating. Rather than judging or criticizing ourselves for succumbing to food cravings, self-compassion encourages us to respond with kindness, understanding, and compassion. It involves recognizing that emotional eating is often a coping mechanism for dealing with difficult emotions and life stressors, and treating ourselves with the same gentleness and care we would offer to a friend in need.

When we practice self-compassion, we acknowledge and validate our feelings without judgment or criticism. We recognize that emotional eating is a natural response to challenging circumstances, and we offer ourselves the support and understanding we need to navigate these emotions. Instead of berating ourselves for turning to food for comfort, we offer ourselves words of encouragement and reassurance, knowing that we are doing the best we can to cope with our emotions.

By practicing self-compassion, we create space for healing and self-acceptance. Rather than trying to suppress or ignore our emotions, we acknowledge them with kindness and compassion, allowing ourselves to experience them fully without judgment. This compassionate approach to emotional eating helps us develop a greater sense of self-awareness and emotional resilience, reducing the need to rely on food for comfort and support.

One way to practice self-compassion is to cultivate a supportive inner dialogue. When we notice ourselves engaging in negative self-talk or self-criticism, we can gently redirect our thoughts with words of kindness and encouragement. We might say to ourselves, "It's okay to be struggling right now. You're doing the best you can, and that's enough." By offering ourselves words of comfort and support, we can soothe our troubled minds and cultivate a greater sense of inner peace and acceptance.

Another way to practice self-compassion is to engage in self-care activities that nourish our body, mind, and soul. This could involve taking a warm bath, going for a walk-in nature, or spending time engaging in a hobby or activity that brings us joy. By prioritizing self-care, we send ourselves the message that we are worthy of love and attention, regardless of our struggles or challenges.

In conclusion, practicing self-compassion is a powerful means of addressing the underlying emotional needs that drive emotional eating. By responding to ourselves with kindness, understanding, and compassion, we create space for healing and self-acceptance. Rather than judging or criticizing ourselves for succumbing to food cravings, we acknowledge and validate our feelings without judgment, allowing ourselves to experience them fully. By cultivating a supportive inner dialogue and engaging in self-care activities that nourish our body, mind, and soul, we can reduce the need to rely on food for emotional comfort and support. With practice and patience, we can develop greater emotional resilience and a healthier relationship with food and our emotions.

Overcoming mental obstacles to weight loss requires a combination of self-awareness, self-compassion, and self-empowerment. By recognizing and challenging negative self-talk, cultivating mindfulness and emotional resilience, and practicing self-compassion and acceptance, you can break free from self-sabotaging patterns and embrace a healthier relationship with food and your body. Remember that change takes time and effort, and be patient and gentle with yourself as you navigate the ups and downs of the weight loss journey. By tapping into your inner strength and resilience, you can overcome obstacles, unleash your full potential, and achieve lasting success in your quest for health and well-being.

CHAPTER 5: NUTRITION BASICS

Nutrition is a cornerstone of any successful weight loss journey. In this chapter, we will explore the fundamentals of nutrition in connection to weight loss, including the role of macronutrients, micronutrients, calorie balance, and dietary strategies for achieving sustainable weight loss.

Understanding Macronutrients: Fueling Your Body
Macronutrients are the three main components of food that provide energy and support various bodily functions: carbohydrates, proteins, and fats.

1. Carbohydrates: Carbohydrates are the body's primary source of energy and are found in foods such as grains, fruits, vegetables, and legumes. When consumed in excess, carbohydrates can contribute to weight gain, especially if they come from refined sources like white bread, sugary snacks, and sweetened beverages. However, complex carbohydrates, such as whole grains, fruits, and vegetables, are rich in fiber, which promotes satiety and helps regulate blood sugar levels, making them a valuable part of a weight loss diet.

2. Proteins: Protein is essential for building and repairing tissues, supporting muscle growth and maintenance, and regulating metabolism. Including protein-rich foods in your diet can help increase feelings of fullness and prevent overeating. Sources of lean protein include poultry, fish, lean cuts of meat, eggs, dairy products, legumes, nuts, and seeds.

3. Fats: Dietary fats are crucial for hormone production, cell membrane integrity, and the absorption of fat-soluble vitamins.

While fats are more calorie-dense than carbohydrates and protein, they also contribute to satiety and help regulate appetite. Healthy sources of fats include avocados, nuts, seeds, olive oil, fatty fish, and coconut oil. Aim to incorporate unsaturated fats, such as monounsaturated and polyunsaturated fats, into your diet while limiting saturated and trans fats.

Calorie Balance: The Key to Weight Loss

At its core, weight loss is about achieving a calorie deficit, where you burn more calories than you consume. This deficit can be achieved through a combination of reducing calorie intake and increasing physical activity.

1. Calorie Intake: To determine your calorie needs for weight loss, you can use online calculators or consult with a registered dietitian. Aim to create a moderate calorie deficit of 500 to 750 calories per day, which can result in a weight loss of about 1 to 1.5 pounds per week. Focus on consuming nutrient-dense foods that provide essential vitamins, minerals, and macronutrients while minimizing empty calories from processed foods, sugary snacks, and high-calorie beverages.

2. Physical Activity: In addition to controlling calorie intake, increasing physical activity is essential for achieving and maintaining weight loss. Aim for at least 150 minutes of moderate-intensity aerobic exercise or 75 minutes of vigorous-intensity exercise per week, along with muscle-strengthening activities on two or more days per week. Incorporate a variety of activities you enjoy, such as walking, jogging, cycling, swimming, dancing, or strength training, to keep your workouts engaging and sustainable.

Micronutrients: Supporting Overall Health

While macronutrients provide energy, micronutrients are essential for supporting overall health and well-being. These include vitamins, minerals, and antioxidants, which play crucial roles in various physiological processes, including metabolism, immune function, and cellular repair.

1. Vitamins: Vitamins are organic compounds that our bodies need in small amounts to function properly. They play key roles in energy production, immune function, and tissue repair. Include a variety of fruits, vegetables, whole grains, lean proteins, and dairy products in your diet to ensure adequate intake of vitamins A, C, D, E, K, and the B-complex vitamins.

2. Minerals: Minerals are inorganic elements that are essential for various physiological functions, including bone health, muscle function, and fluid balance. Common minerals include calcium, magnesium, potassium, sodium, iron, zinc, and selenium. Aim to include a diverse array of nutrient-rich foods in your diet to meet your mineral needs, including leafy greens, nuts, seeds, whole grains, lean meats, and dairy products.

Dietary Strategies for Weight Loss Success

In addition to understanding the role of macronutrients, calorie balance, and micronutrients, several dietary strategies can support weight loss success:

1. Portion Control: Be mindful of portion sizes and avoid overeating by using smaller plates, measuring serving sizes, and paying attention to hunger and fullness cues.

2. Meal Planning and Preparation: Plan and prepare meals in advance to ensure that you have nutritious options readily available and avoid relying on convenience foods or takeout meals.

3. Mindful Eating: Practice mindful eating by slowing down, savoring each bite, and paying attention to hunger and fullness signals. This can help prevent overeating and promote greater satisfaction with meals.

4. Hydration: Stay hydrated by drinking plenty of water throughout the day. Sometimes thirst can be mistaken for hunger, leading to unnecessary snacking or overeating.

5. Balanced Diet: Aim for a balanced diet that includes a variety of nutrient-dense foods from all food groups, including fruits, vegetables, whole grains, lean proteins, and healthy fats.

In conclusion, understanding the fundamentals of nutrition is essential for achieving and maintaining weight loss success. By focusing on macronutrients, calorie balance, and micronutrients, as well as incorporating dietary strategies for weight loss, you can create a sustainable approach to eating that supports your health and well-being. Remember to consult with a healthcare professional or registered dietitian before making significant changes to your diet or exercise routine, especially if you have any underlying health conditions or concerns. With dedication, consistency, and a focus on balanced nutrition, you can achieve your weight loss goals and enjoy a healthier, happier lifestyle.

Now let us take a deeper look at balanced diet and portion control as they are foundational principles of healthy eating that play crucial roles in supporting overall health, managing weight, and reducing the risk of chronic diseases. In this chapter, we will explore the significance of a balanced diet and portion control, their impact on health outcomes, and practical strategies for incorporating these principles into your daily life.

Understanding a Balanced Diet

A balanced diet is one that provides the body with all the essential nutrients it needs to function optimally while maintaining energy balance. This means consuming a variety of foods from all the major food groups in appropriate proportions to ensure adequate intake of essential nutrients.

1. **Nutrient Variety**: Each food group contributes unique nutrients to the diet, including carbohydrates, proteins, fats, vitamins, minerals, and antioxidants. By incorporating a variety of foods from different food groups into your meals and snacks, you can ensure that your body receives a wide range of nutrients necessary for growth, development, and overall health.

2. **Macronutrient Balance**: A balanced diet includes appropriate proportions of carbohydrates, proteins, and fats. Carbohydrates provide the body with energy, while proteins are essential for building and repairing tissues, and fats are necessary for hormone production and nutrient absorption. Balancing these macronutrients helps regulate blood sugar levels, support muscle growth and repair, and promote satiety and satisfaction with meals.

3. **Micronutrient Adequacy**: In addition to macronutrients, a balanced diet ensures adequate intake of vitamins and minerals, which play crucial roles in various physiological processes,

including metabolism, immune function, and cellular repair. Consuming a diverse array of nutrient-rich foods, such as fruits, vegetables, whole grains, lean proteins, and dairy products, helps meet micronutrient needs and support overall health and well-being.

The Impact of a Balanced Diet on Health

A balanced diet has far-reaching implications for health outcomes, influencing everything from energy levels and mood to disease risk and longevity. Here are some of the key ways in which a balanced diet supports overall health:

1. Weight Management: A balanced diet helps regulate energy balance, ensuring that you consume the appropriate number of calories to support your activity level and metabolic needs. By choosing nutrient-dense foods and controlling portion sizes, you can achieve and maintain a healthy weight, reducing the risk of obesity and related health conditions.

2. Nutrient Absorption: Consuming a variety of nutrient-rich foods ensures adequate intake of vitamins and minerals necessary for optimal health. Certain nutrients, such as vitamin C and iron, enhance the absorption of others, ensuring efficient nutrient utilization and supporting overall health and vitality.

3. Disease Prevention: A balanced diet rich in fruits, vegetables, whole grains, lean proteins, and healthy fats provides essential nutrients and antioxidants that help reduce the risk of chronic diseases, including heart disease, diabetes, cancer, and obesity. These foods are rich in fiber, vitamins, and phytochemicals that support immune function, reduce inflammation, and promote overall well-being.

4. Energy and Vitality: The foods we eat provide the fuel our bodies need to function optimally. A balanced diet provides a steady supply of energy to support physical activity, mental clarity, and emotional well-being, helping you feel energized and vital throughout the day.

The Role of Portion Control

While eating a balanced diet is important for overall health, portion control is equally crucial for managing weight and preventing overeating. Portion control involves being mindful of portion sizes and avoiding consuming larger portions than your body needs.

1. Calorie Awareness: Portion control helps you become more aware of the number of calories you consume, making it easier to maintain energy balance and achieve weight loss or weight maintenance goals. By controlling portion sizes, you can prevent excess calorie intake and avoid weight gain.

2. Satiety and Satisfaction: Eating appropriate portion sizes helps regulate appetite and promote feelings of satiety and satisfaction with meals. By consuming smaller portions of nutrient-dense foods, you can feel full and satisfied while still enjoying a variety of flavors and textures.

3. Preventing Overeating: Portion control helps prevent overeating by limiting the amount of food you consume at each meal or snack. By being mindful of portion sizes and listening to hunger and fullness cues, you can avoid eating past the point of satisfaction and reduce the risk of weight gain.

Strategies for Balancing Your Diet and Controlling Portions
Incorporating a balanced diet and portion control into your daily life doesn't have to be complicated. Here are some practical strategies to help you achieve a healthy balance:

1. Fill Half Your Plate with Fruits and Vegetables: Aim to fill half your plate with fruits and vegetables at each meal. These foods are low in calories and rich in vitamins, minerals, and fiber, helping you feel full and satisfied while supporting overall health.

2. Choose Whole Grains: Opt for whole grains, such as brown rice, quinoa, oats, and whole wheat bread and pasta, over refined grains. Whole grains are higher in fiber and nutrients, providing sustained energy and promoting feelings of fullness.

3. Include Lean Proteins: Incorporate lean protein sources, such as poultry, fish, tofu, beans, and lentils, into your meals and snacks. Protein helps regulate appetite, supports muscle growth and repair, and promotes satiety and satisfaction with meals.

4. Practice Mindful Eating: Slow down and savor each bite, paying attention to hunger and fullness cues. Eat slowly, chew thoroughly, and pause between bites to check in with your body's hunger and fullness signals.

5. Use Smaller Plates and Bowls: Serve meals and snacks on smaller plates and bowls to visually reduce portion sizes. This can help trick your brain into feeling satisfied with smaller portions, even if you're eating the same amount of food.

6. Portion Out Snacks: Instead of eating directly from the package, portion out snacks into individual servings to prevent mindless eating and control portion sizes.

7. Listen to Your Body: Pay attention to your body's hunger and fullness cues, eating when you're hungry and stopping when you're satisfied. Avoid eating out of boredom, stress, or other emotional triggers.

In summary, a balanced diet and portion control are essential components of a healthy eating pattern that supports overall health, weight management, and disease prevention. By consuming a variety of nutrient-dense foods from all food groups in appropriate portions, you can ensure adequate intake of essential nutrients while controlling calorie intake and maintaining energy balance. Incorporate practical strategies for balancing your diet and controlling portions into your daily life to support your health and well-being for years to come. Remember that small changes add up over time, so focus on progress, not perfection, and celebrate your successes along the way. With dedication, consistency, and a commitment to healthful eating habits, you can achieve and maintain a balanced diet and enjoy the benefits of optimal nutrition.

CHAPTER 6: BUILDING HEALTHY HABITS

Embarking on a weight loss journey can feel daunting, but incorporating healthy habits into your daily life can make the process more manageable and sustainable. In this chapter, we'll explore practical tips and strategies for integrating healthy habits into your routine to support weight loss and improve overall well-being.

1. Set Realistic Goals

In the realm of weight loss, the importance of setting realistic and attainable goals cannot be overstated. Rather than fixating on rapid, drastic weight reduction, prioritize gradual and sustainable lifestyle adjustments. Begin by establishing small, manageable objectives that can be pursued daily or weekly. These may include incrementally boosting your daily step count, incorporating an additional serving of vegetables into your meals, or curbing your consumption of sugary beverages. Each achievement, no matter how minor, deserves celebration, serving as a motivating force to propel you forward. Be flexible and prepared to adapt your goals as circumstances evolve, ensuring that your trajectory remains aligned with your aspirations. By adhering to this approach, you foster a sense of empowerment and resilience, laying the groundwork for enduring success on your weight loss journey.

2. Prioritize Nutrition

Nutrition plays a central role in weight loss and overall health. Focus on nourishing your body with nutrient-dense foods that provide essential vitamins, minerals, and macronutrients. Aim to fill your plate with a variety of fruits, vegetables, whole grains, lean proteins, and healthy fats at each meal. Experiment with new recipes and cooking techniques to keep meals exciting and satisfying. Planning and preparing meals in advance can also help you stay on track with your nutritional goals and avoid relying on unhealthy convenience foods.

3. Practice Portion Control

Ensuring effective portion control is pivotal in managing calorie consumption and facilitating weight loss endeavors. Remain conscientious of portion sizes, steering clear of oversized servings, particularly when dining out or partaking in packaged foods. Employing smaller plates, bowls, and utensils serves as an effective strategy to regulate portion sizes and deter overindulgence. Cultivate an awareness of your body's hunger and fullness signals, adopting a deliberate approach to eating by savoring each bite and pausing when a sense of satisfaction is attained, rather than allowing yourself to become uncomfortably full. Embrace the notion that it's perfectly acceptable to leave food uneaten on your plate if satiety has been achieved, and refrain from seeking solace in food when faced with boredom or emotional triggers. By mastering the art of portion control and mindful eating, you empower yourself to navigate mealtimes with greater self-awareness and discretion, thereby fostering a healthier relationship with food and promoting successful weight management.

4. Stay Hydrated

Maintaining proper hydration levels is paramount for overall well-being and can significantly aid in weight loss endeavors. Water intake plays a crucial role in inducing feelings of satiety, preventing overeating, and averting dehydration. Strive to consume a minimum of 8 glasses of water daily, adjusting this amount as needed based on factors such as physical activity levels and environmental conditions, particularly in hot climates. Embrace the habit of carrying a reusable water bottle with you throughout the day, facilitating easy access to hydration wherever you go. By prioritizing hydration and opting for water over sugary beverages or snacks in response to thirst cues, you not only support your weight loss goals but also promote optimal hydration and overall health. Cultivate mindfulness regarding your body's hydration needs, making a conscious effort to maintain adequate fluid intake as an integral component of your daily routine.

5. Move Your Body Regularly

Engaging in regular physical activity is indispensable for achieving weight loss goals, given its multifaceted benefits that extend beyond calorie burning. Physical exercise not only aids in calorie expenditure but also facilitates the development of lean muscle mass, thereby contributing to improved metabolic function and overall fitness levels. Identify activities that resonate with your interests and preferences, whether it's walking, jogging, cycling, swimming, dancing, or strength training, and integrate them seamlessly into your daily routine. Strive to adhere to established guidelines recommending at least 150 minutes of moderate-intensity aerobic exercise or 75 minutes of vigorous-intensity exercise per week, complemented by muscle-strengthening activities on two or more days.

Embrace opportunities to incorporate physical activity into your everyday life, such as opting for the stairs instead of the elevator, parking farther away from your destination to necessitate walking, or interspersing brief bursts of activity throughout your day. By embracing a holistic approach to physical activity and integrating movement into your daily routine, you pave the way for enhanced weight loss outcomes and improved overall health and well-being.

6. Get Adequate Sleep

Prioritizing sufficient sleep is paramount not only for weight loss but also for overall health and well-being. Strive to achieve between 7-9 hours of uninterrupted sleep each night to facilitate proper hormone regulation, metabolism, and appetite control. Establishing a consistent sleep schedule, whereby you retire and awaken at the same times daily, aids in regulating your body's internal clock and optimizing sleep quality, even on weekends. Cultivate a calming bedtime routine to signal to your body that it's time to unwind and prepare for restorative sleep.

Consider activities such as taking a warm bath, reading a book, or practicing relaxation techniques like deep breathing or meditation to promote relaxation and reduce stress levels. Prior to bedtime, refrain from consuming caffeine or alcohol, as well as engaging with electronic devices, as these factors can disrupt your ability to fall asleep and diminish sleep quality. By embracing these strategies and prioritizing sleep hygiene, you foster an environment conducive to restful sleep and support your weight loss efforts and overall health in the process.

7. Manage Stress

Chronic stress poses a significant threat to weight loss endeavors, as it can precipitate various detrimental effects on both physical and mental well-being. Stress triggers emotional eating, leading to the consumption of comfort foods that are often high in calories and low in nutritional value. Moreover, stress disrupts sleep patterns, compromising the body's ability to recover and regulate metabolic processes. Elevated cortisol levels, a hallmark of chronic stress, further exacerbate weight gain by promoting fat accumulation, particularly around the abdominal region.

To counteract the deleterious effects of stress on weight loss, it's imperative to adopt effective stress management techniques. Incorporate practices such as deep breathing, meditation, yoga, or progressive muscle relaxation into your daily routine to alleviate stress and induce a state of calmness and relaxation. Additionally, prioritize engaging in self-care activities that foster joy and relaxation, such as spending quality time with loved ones, pursuing hobbies, or immersing yourself in nature. If stress persists and becomes overwhelming, don't hesitate to seek professional support from a therapist or counselor who can provide guidance and strategies for coping with stress and emotional challenges effectively. By addressing stress proactively and implementing stress-reducing practices, you can bolster your resilience and enhance your capacity to navigate the challenges of weight loss with greater ease and success.

8. Practice Mindful Eating

Mindful eating is a transformative practice that fosters a deeper connection with food and cultivates a greater awareness of one's body and its signals. It entails immersing oneself fully in the present moment, free from judgment or distraction, and savoring each morsel with intentionality and appreciation. By slowing down and deliberately engaging with the sensory experience of eating, individuals can heighten their awareness of the taste, texture, and aroma of their food, thereby deriving greater pleasure and satisfaction from each bite.

Central to mindful eating is the cultivation of attunement to the body's hunger and fullness cues, allowing individuals to eat in accordance with their physiological needs rather than external influences. By honoring these cues and eating when genuinely hungry while stopping when comfortably satisfied, individuals can foster a harmonious relationship with food and promote optimal nourishment and well-being.

Crucially, mindful eating entails avoiding distractions during meals, such as watching television or scrolling on electronic devices, as these behaviors can disrupt the mindful eating experience and lead to mindless consumption of calories. By committing to being fully present and attentive during meals, individuals can harness the transformative power of mindful eating to cultivate a more balanced and fulfilling relationship with food, promoting greater satisfaction, and supporting weight loss efforts in the process.

9. Seek Support

Embarking on a weight loss journey is undoubtedly daunting, but it's important to remember that you need not face it alone. Drawing upon the support and encouragement of others can be instrumental in maintaining motivation and momentum throughout your journey. Seek out friends, family members, or a supportive community who can offer guidance, empathy, and accountability as you navigate the challenges of weight loss. Additionally, consider enlisting the expertise of healthcare professionals such as registered dietitians, personal trainers, or health coaches, who can provide tailored advice and support to help you achieve your goals.

It's essential to recognize that progress in weight loss is not always linear, and setbacks are a natural part of the process. Instead of becoming discouraged by obstacles, practice self-compassion and acknowledge the progress you've made, no matter how small. Celebrate your successes, however modest they may seem, and use setbacks as opportunities for growth and learning. By cultivating a supportive network and adopting a compassionate mindset, you can navigate the ups and downs of your weight loss journey with resilience and determination.

Incorporating healthy habits into your daily life is essential for achieving and maintaining weight loss. By setting realistic goals, prioritizing nutrition, practicing portion control, staying hydrated, moving your body regularly, getting adequate sleep, managing stress, practicing mindful eating, and seeking support, you can create a sustainable approach to weight loss that supports your overall health and well-being. Remember that small changes add up over time, so focus on progress, not perfection, and celebrate your successes along the way. With dedication, consistency, and a positive mindset, you can achieve your weight loss goals and enjoy a healthier, happier lifestyle.

CHAPTER 7: EXERCISE AND PHYSICAL ACTIVITY

Exercise is a fundamental component of any successful weight loss journey, playing a pivotal role in achieving and maintaining a healthy body weight. In this chapter, we'll delve into the multifaceted benefits of exercise for weight loss, explore different types of exercise modalities, and provide practical tips for incorporating exercise into your daily routine.

Understanding the Benefits of Exercise for Weight Loss

Exercise offers a myriad of benefits beyond simply burning calories. It enhances metabolic rate, promotes fat loss, preserves lean muscle mass, and improves overall physical fitness and health. Regular exercise can also have positive effects on mood, energy levels, and motivation, making it easier to adhere to a healthy lifestyle and dietary habits.

One of the key mechanisms through which exercise facilitates weight loss is by increasing energy expenditure. When you engage in physical activity, your body burns calories to fuel muscular contractions and support various physiological processes. Over time, this calorie expenditure contributes to a negative energy balance, where you burn more calories than you consume, leading to weight loss.

Moreover, exercise can help shift your body composition by reducing body fat percentage while preserving lean muscle mass. This is particularly important for maintaining metabolic rate, as muscle tissue is more metabolically active than fat tissue, meaning it burns more calories at rest.

Types of Exercise Modalities

There are various types of exercise modalities, each offering unique benefits and catering to different preferences and fitness levels. Some popular options include:

1. Cardiovascular Exercise: Cardiovascular or aerobic exercise involves activities that elevate your heart rate and increase oxygen consumption, such as walking, running, cycling, swimming, and dancing. Cardiovascular exercise is effective for burning calories, improving cardiovascular health, and enhancing endurance.

2. Strength Training: Strength training, also known as resistance training or weightlifting, involves using external resistance, such as free weights, resistance bands, or weight machines, to challenge your muscles. Strength training helps build and maintain lean muscle mass, which is essential for metabolic health and weight management.

3. Flexibility and Mobility Exercises: Flexibility and mobility exercises, including stretching, yoga, and Pilates, focus on improving joint range of motion, flexibility, and overall mobility. These exercises can complement cardiovascular and strength training workouts, enhance recovery, and reduce the risk of injury.

4. High-Intensity Interval Training (HIIT): HIIT involves alternating between short bursts of high-intensity exercise and periods of rest or lower-intensity activity. HIIT workouts are time-efficient and effective for burning calories, improving cardiovascular fitness, and boosting metabolism.

Practical Tips for Incorporating Exercise into Your Routine
Incorporating exercise into your daily routine doesn't have to be complicated or overwhelming. Here are some practical tips to help you get started and stay motivated:

1. Set Realistic Goals: Start by setting realistic and achievable exercise goals based on your current fitness level and lifestyle. Gradually increase the intensity, duration, and frequency of your workouts as you progress.

2. Find Activities You Enjoy: Choose activities that you enjoy and look forward to, whether it's dancing, hiking, playing sports, or attending group fitness classes. Enjoying your workouts increases adherence and makes exercise feel less like a chore.

3. Schedule Exercise Sessions: Treat exercise like any other important appointment by scheduling regular workout sessions into your calendar. Consistency is key to seeing results and forming lasting habits.

4. Mix It Up: Keep your workouts interesting and challenging by incorporating a variety of exercise modalities and activities. Try new workouts, classes, or outdoor activities to prevent boredom and plateaus.

5. Listen to Your Body: Pay attention to your body's signals and adjust your workouts accordingly. Rest when needed, and don't push through pain or discomfort. Consistent, gradual progress is more sustainable than pushing yourself too hard and risking injury.

6. Stay Hydrated and Fuel Your Body: Drink plenty of water before, during, and after exercise to stay hydrated. Eat a balanced meal or snack containing carbohydrates and protein before workouts to fuel your body and support recovery afterward.

7. Track Your Progress: Keep track of your workouts, progress, and achievements to stay motivated and accountable. Use a fitness journal, smartphone app, or wearable fitness tracker to monitor your activity levels, set goals, and celebrate milestones.

Exercise is an essential component of weight loss, offering numerous physical, mental, and emotional benefits. By incorporating a variety of exercise modalities into your routine, setting realistic goals, staying consistent, and listening to your body, you can achieve sustainable weight loss and improve your overall health and well-being. Remember that exercise should be enjoyable and fulfilling, so choose activities that you love and make fitness a lifelong journey. With dedication, perseverance, and a positive mindset, you can reach your weight loss goals and enjoy a healthier, more active lifestyle.

However, designing an effective exercise routine is essential for achieving your fitness goals, whether they involve weight loss, muscle gain, improved endurance, or overall health and well-being. In this chapter, we'll provide comprehensive guidance on creating a personalized exercise plan that is tailored to your needs, preferences, and fitness level.

Assessing Your Goals and Needs

Before you can design an exercise routine, it's crucial to clarify your goals and assess your individual needs. Ask yourself:

1. What are my fitness goals? (e.g., weight loss, muscle gain, improved cardiovascular health)

2. What is my current fitness level and experience with exercise?

3. What are my preferences and interests when it comes to physical activity?

4. Do I have any specific limitations or health concerns that need to be considered?

By understanding your objectives and considering your unique circumstances, you can create a workout plan that is both effective and sustainable.

Designing Your Exercise Routine

Once you've identified your goals and selected the components of your exercise routine, it's time to design your plan. Consider the following factors:

1. **Frequency**: How often will you exercise each week? Aim for a minimum of 3-5 days per week, with at least one rest day for recovery.

2. **Duration**: How long will each workout session last? Aim for a total of 150-300 minutes of moderate-intensity aerobic exercise per week, along with 2-3 sessions of strength training.

3. **Intensity**: How hard will you work during your workouts? Adjust the intensity of your workouts based on your fitness

level and goals. Incorporate both moderate-intensity and high-intensity exercise sessions for optimal results.

4. **Progression**: How will you progress and challenge yourself over time? Gradually increase the duration, intensity, or complexity of your workouts as you become fitter and stronger.

5. **Variety**: How will you keep your workouts interesting and engaging? Incorporate a variety of exercises, activities, and workout formats to prevent boredom and plateauing.

Sample Exercise Routine

Here's an example of a well-rounded exercise routine that incorporates the components discussed above:

1. Monday: Strength Training (Full-Body Workout)

- Squats: 3 sets of 10 reps
- Push-Ups: 3 sets of 10 reps
- Bent-Over Rows: 3 sets of 10 reps
- Lunges: 3 sets of 10 reps (each leg)
- Plank: 3 sets of 30 seconds

2. Tuesday: Cardiovascular Exercise

- 30 minutes of brisk walking or jogging

3. Wednesday: Rest or Active Recovery (Yoga or Stretching)

4. Thursday: Strength Training (Upper Body)

- Bench Press: 3 sets of 10 reps
- Pull-Ups or Lat Pulldowns: 3 sets of 10 reps
- Shoulder Press: 3 sets of 10 reps
- Bicep Curls: 3 sets of 10 reps
- Triceps Dips: 3 sets of 10 reps

5. Friday: Cardiovascular Exercise

- 30 minutes of cycling or swimming

6. Saturday: Flexibility and Mobility Exercises

- 20 minutes of yoga or stretching

7. Sunday: Active Rest (Walking, Hiking, or Recreational Activity)

Tips for Success

To make your exercise routine more effective and sustainable, consider the following tips:

1. **Start Slowly and Progress Gradually**: Ease into your exercise routine to prevent injury and burnout. Gradually increase the intensity and duration of your workouts as you become more comfortable and confident.

2. **Listen to Your Body**: Pay attention to how your body responds to exercise and adjust your routine accordingly. Rest when needed, and don't push through pain or discomfort.

3. **Stay Consistent**: Consistency is key to seeing results. Stick to your exercise routine as much as possible, even when life gets busy or challenging.

4. **Mix It Up**: Keep your workouts interesting and prevent boredom by incorporating a variety of exercises, activities, and workout formats into your routine.

5. **Stay Hydrated and Fuel Your Body**: Drink plenty of water before, during, and after exercise to stay hydrated. Eat a balanced diet rich in nutrients to fuel your workouts and support recovery.

6. **Monitor Your Progress**: Keep track of your workouts, progress, and achievements to stay motivated and accountable. Celebrate your successes and milestones along the way.

Creating an effective exercise routine requires careful planning, consideration of your goals and needs, and a commitment to consistency and progression. By incorporating a variety of exercise modalities, designing a well-rounded workout plan, and adhering to best practices for success, you can achieve your fitness goals and enjoy the numerous benefits of regular physical activity. Remember to listen to your body, stay flexible and adaptable, and above all, have fun with your workouts. With dedication and determination, you can create a sustainable exercise routine that supports your health and well-being for years to come.

CHAPTER 8: SLEEP AND WEIGHT LOSS

Sleep plays a crucial role in overall health and well-being, with emerging research highlighting its significance in the context of weight management and weight loss. In this chapter, we'll explore the intricate relationship between sleep and weight, delve into the mechanisms underlying this connection, and provide practical tips for optimizing sleep to support your weight loss goals.

Understanding the Link Between Sleep and Weight

Research suggests that insufficient or poor-quality sleep is associated with weight gain and obesity. Numerous studies have demonstrated a clear correlation between shorter sleep duration and increased body weight, as well as a higher risk of obesity and metabolic disorders.

Several factors contribute to this relationship:

1. **Hormonal Regulation**: Sleep plays a critical role in regulating hormones that influence appetite, hunger, and satiety. Sleep deprivation disrupts the balance of key hormones, such as leptin and ghrelin, which can lead to increased appetite, cravings for high-calorie foods, and decreased feelings of fullness.

2. **Metabolic Function**: Adequate sleep is essential for maintaining optimal metabolic function, including glucose metabolism and insulin sensitivity. Sleep deprivation can impair glucose regulation and insulin sensitivity, increasing the risk of insulin resistance, metabolic syndrome, and type 2 diabetes.

3. **Energy Balance**: Sleep influences energy balance by affecting both energy intake (calories consumed) and energy expenditure (calories burned). Sleep-deprived individuals may consume more calories, particularly from unhealthy, high-calorie foods, while also experiencing reduced energy expenditure and physical activity levels.

Mechanisms Behind the Sleep-Weight Connection
Several physiological mechanisms underlie the relationship between sleep and weight:

1. **Appetite Regulation**: Sleep deprivation disrupts the normal regulation of appetite hormones, leading to increased hunger and cravings for calorie-dense foods. Leptin, the hormone responsible for signaling satiety, decreases with insufficient sleep, while ghrelin, the hormone that stimulates appetite, increases.

2. **Reward Pathways**: Sleep deprivation alters brain activity in regions associated with reward processing and decision-making, making individuals more susceptible to food cues and cravings for unhealthy, high-calorie foods. This can contribute to overeating and weight gain over time.

3. **Metabolic Dysregulation**: Chronic sleep deprivation disrupts metabolic function, leading to alterations in glucose metabolism, insulin sensitivity, and lipid metabolism. These changes can predispose individuals to weight gain, insulin resistance, and metabolic disorders.

Practical Strategies for Improving Sleep Quality

Optimizing sleep quality is essential for supporting weight loss efforts and overall health. Here are some practical strategies to enhance sleep quality:

1. **Establish a Consistent Sleep Schedule**: Consistency is key when it comes to regulating your body's internal clock and promoting better sleep quality. Aim to maintain a consistent sleep schedule by going to bed and waking up at the same time each day, including weekends. This helps synchronize your body's circadian rhythm, making it easier to fall asleep and wake up naturally. By sticking to a regular sleep-wake routine, you can optimize the quality and duration of your sleep, leading to improved overall health and well-being.

2. **Create a Relaxing Bedtime Routine**: Creating a soothing bedtime routine is essential for preparing your body and mind for sleep. Engage in calming activities that signal to your body it's time to wind down, such as reading a book, taking a warm bath, or practicing relaxation techniques like deep breathing or meditation. These activities can help reduce stress and anxiety, quiet the mind, and promote relaxation, making it easier to transition into sleep. Additionally, listening to soothing music or gentle nature sounds can further enhance the relaxation process and create a peaceful sleep environment. By incorporating these calming bedtime rituals into your nightly routine, you can improve sleep quality and overall well-being.

3. **Create a Sleep-Friendly Environment**: Creating an optimal sleep environment is crucial for promoting restful and uninterrupted sleep. Ensure your bedroom is conducive to sleep by maintaining a cool, dark, and quiet atmosphere. Invest in a high-quality mattress and pillows that provide adequate support and comfort for your body. Additionally, minimize distractions such as electronic devices, excess noise, and bright lights that can disrupt sleep. Consider using blackout curtains or eye masks to block out external light sources, and use white noise machines or earplugs to drown out any disruptive sounds. By creating a peaceful and comfortable sleep environment, you can enhance sleep quality and wake up feeling refreshed and rejuvenated each morning.

4. **Limit Caffeine and Stimulants**: To promote better sleep quality, it's essential to limit your intake of caffeine and other stimulants, especially in the afternoon and evening hours. Caffeine, found in beverages like coffee, tea, and energy drinks, can interfere with your body's ability to relax and fall asleep, disrupting your natural sleep-wake cycle. Consuming these stimulants too close to bedtime can result in difficulty falling asleep, as well as fragmented and restless sleep throughout the night. Instead, opt for caffeine-free alternatives such as herbal tea or decaffeinated beverages in the hours leading up to bedtime. By reducing your intake of caffeine and stimulants in the evening, you can support your body's natural sleep processes and enjoy more restorative and rejuvenating sleep.

5. **Limit Screen Time Before Bed**: To improve sleep quality, it's important to limit exposure to electronic devices before

bedtime. The blue light emitted by smartphones, tablets, computers, and other screens can disrupt your body's production of melatonin, a hormone that regulates sleep-wake cycles. Excessive exposure to blue light in the evening can suppress melatonin levels, making it harder to fall asleep and potentially affecting the quality of your sleep. To minimize the impact of electronic devices on your sleep, establish a "screen curfew" at least an hour before bedtime. During this time, engage in relaxing activities such as reading a book, practicing meditation, or listening to calming music. Additionally, consider using blue light-blocking glasses or installing apps that reduce blue light emission on electronic devices to further mitigate the effects of screen exposure on your sleep. By reducing screen time before bed, you can promote better sleep hygiene and improve overall sleep quality.

6. **Exercise Regularly**: Regular physical activity is beneficial for sleep quality, but timing is key. Engage in moderate exercise earlier in the day to promote better sleep quality, as it can help regulate your sleep-wake cycle and reduce stress. However, avoid vigorous exercise close to bedtime, as it can stimulate your body and make it difficult to fall asleep. Vigorous activities raise your heart rate and body temperature, which may interfere with your ability to relax and unwind before bed. Instead, opt for calming activities in the evening, such as gentle stretching or yoga, to prepare your body for sleep. By incorporating regular exercise into your daily routine and timing it appropriately, you can improve sleep quality and enjoy more restful nights.

7. **Manage Stress and Anxiety**: To enhance sleep quality, incorporate stress-reduction techniques into your bedtime routine. Mindfulness meditation, progressive muscle relaxation, and journaling are effective strategies for alleviating stress and anxiety that may interfere with sleep. Mindfulness meditation involves focusing on the present moment and letting go of racing thoughts, promoting relaxation and calmness. Progressive muscle relaxation entails tensing and then releasing muscle groups to reduce physical tension and promote relaxation throughout the body. Journaling allows you to express your thoughts and feelings, helping to clear your mind before bedtime and alleviate stress. By practicing these stress-reduction techniques regularly, you can create a sense of calm and relaxation that prepares your body and mind for restful sleep. Incorporate these practices into your nightly routine to promote better sleep and wake up feeling refreshed and rejuvenated each morning.

Sleep plays a critical role in weight management and weight loss, influencing appetite regulation, metabolic function, and energy balance. Chronic sleep deprivation can disrupt hormonal regulation, impair metabolic function, and increase the risk of weight gain and obesity. By prioritizing sleep and implementing strategies to improve sleep quality, you can support your weight loss goals and promote overall health and well-being. Incorporate healthy sleep habits into your daily routine, create a conducive sleep environment, and address any underlying sleep disorders or disturbances to optimize your sleep quality and enhance your weight loss efforts. With adequate, restorative sleep, you can improve your chances of achieving sustainable weight loss and enjoying a healthier, happier life.

CHAPTER 9: SOCIAL SUPPORT AND ACCOUNTABILITY

Embarking on a weight loss journey can be a challenging endeavor, filled with ups and downs, triumphs, and setbacks. In the midst of this journey, having a support system can make all the difference, providing encouragement, accountability, and motivation to help you stay on track and achieve your goals. In this chapter, we'll explore the importance of having a support system in your weight loss journey and how it can enhance your chances of success.

1. Emotional Support

Embarking on a weight loss journey is often accompanied by a rollercoaster of emotions. Initially, there's the excitement and determination fueled by the prospect of positive change and improved health. However, as the journey progresses, challenges inevitably arise, and feelings of frustration, self-doubt, and even despair may surface.

During these trying times, having a support system in place can be invaluable. Whether it's comprised of friends, family members, or an online community, the presence of individuals who understand and empathize with your struggles can provide a much-needed source of comfort and encouragement. They serve as a pillar of support, offering reassurance and guidance when you find yourself facing obstacles or doubting your abilities.

One of the most significant benefits of emotional support is its ability to buoy your spirits during moments of adversity. When you hit a plateau in your weight loss journey or encounter setbacks, having someone to lean on can make all the difference. They can offer words of encouragement, remind you of how far you've come, and provide perspective when your own vision becomes clouded by self-doubt.

Furthermore, emotional support can be instrumental in celebrating your victories, no matter how small. Whether you've reached a milestone weight loss goal, conquered a challenging workout, or resisted temptation in the face of cravings, having someone to share your achievements with can amplify the joy and satisfaction of your accomplishments. Their genuine enthusiasm and pride in your progress serve as powerful reminders of your strength and resilience, motivating you to continue pushing forward.

Additionally, emotional support fosters a sense of camaraderie and shared purpose, as you navigate the highs and lows of your weight loss journey together. By surrounding yourself with individuals who share your goals and aspirations, you create a supportive community that understands the challenges you face and celebrates your successes alongside you. This sense of solidarity strengthens your resolve and provides a sense of belonging, reinforcing your commitment to your health and well-being.

In essence, emotional support acts as a lifeline, helping you navigate the unpredictable terrain of your weight loss journey with greater resilience and positivity. Whether it's a shoulder to lean on during difficult times or a cheerleader to celebrate your victories, having a support system in place can make the difference between giving up and pressing on. So, cultivate and nurture your support system, lean on them when needed, and be open to offering support in return. Together, you can overcome obstacles, celebrate successes, and create a healthier, happier life.

2. Accountability

Accountability is a powerful force in achieving success, especially when it comes to weight loss goals. A support system can provide the necessary framework for this accountability, serving as a valuable partner in your journey towards better health and fitness.

One of the primary functions of an accountability partner within your support system is to hold you to your commitments and goals. When you share your aspirations with others, whether it's a workout buddy, a friend, or a family member, you create a sense of responsibility to follow through on your plans. Knowing that someone is rooting for you and expecting you to make progress can serve as a powerful motivator to stay disciplined and focused, even when faced with challenges or setbacks.

For example, having a workout buddy who holds you accountable for showing up at the gym can significantly increase your adherence to an exercise routine. When you know that your friend is counting on you to be there, you're more likely to prioritize your workouts and make them a consistent part of your schedule. Similarly, having a friend or family member who checks in on your progress regularly can provide an added layer of accountability, helping you stay on track and avoid slipping back into old habits.

Moreover, accountability partners can offer support and encouragement when you need it most. They can celebrate your successes with you, offer words of encouragement during challenging times, and provide a listening ear when you're feeling discouraged. Knowing that you have someone in your corner who believes in you and your ability to succeed can boost your confidence and motivation, making it easier to overcome obstacles and stay committed to your weight loss goals.

In addition to providing emotional support and encouragement, accountability partners can also offer practical assistance and guidance to help you stay on track. They can help you set realistic goals, create action plans, and track your progress over time. By regularly reviewing your goals and progress with your accountability partner, you can identify areas where you may need to adjust your approach or make changes to your routine to stay on course.

Overall, having an accountability partner within your support system can be instrumental in helping you achieve your weight loss goals. Whether it's a workout buddy, a friend, or a family member, having someone to hold you accountable, provide support and encouragement, and offer practical guidance can significantly increase your chances of success. So, don't hesitate to reach out to those around you and enlist their support in your journey towards better health and fitness. Together, you can achieve more than you ever thought possible.

3. Practical Support

In the pursuit of weight loss goals, practical assistance from a support system can be instrumental in overcoming obstacles and facilitating progress. While emotional support and accountability are crucial aspects of a support network, practical assistance adds another layer of support by addressing logistical challenges and providing tangible help to ease the burden of your weight loss journey.

One significant way in which a support system can offer practical assistance is through meal prep and nutrition guidance. Planning and preparing healthy meals can be time-consuming and daunting, especially for individuals juggling busy schedules and other responsibilities. However, with the help of friends, family members, or even professional nutritionists, you can streamline the process and ensure that your meals align with your weight loss goals. Whether it's sharing recipes, grocery shopping together, or preparing meals in advance, having assistance in meal prep can make healthy eating more accessible and sustainable.

Similarly, support system members can provide valuable guidance and support in structuring an effective workout routine. Whether you're new to exercise or looking to switch up your fitness regimen, having someone with experience and knowledge to offer advice can be invaluable. They can help you create a customized workout plan tailored to your goals and preferences, provide instruction on proper form and technique, and offer encouragement to stay consistent with your workouts. Additionally, having a workout buddy to join you in your fitness endeavors can make exercise more enjoyable and motivating.

Beyond meal prep and workout guidance, practical assistance from a support system can also extend to other areas of your life that may impact your ability to prioritize your health and well-being. For instance, if you're a parent, childcare support from family members or trusted caregivers can free up time for you to focus on self-care activities like exercise or meal planning. Likewise, assistance with household chores or errands can help alleviate stress and create space in your schedule for healthy habits.

By enlisting the help of others, you can lighten your load and remove barriers that might otherwise hinder your progress in your weight loss journey. This collaborative approach allows you to focus more fully on your health and well-being, knowing that you have a support system to lean on for practical assistance and guidance. Additionally, involving others in your journey fosters a sense of teamwork and camaraderie, strengthening the bonds of your support network and enhancing your overall success.

In conclusion, practical assistance from a support system plays a vital role in making your weight loss journey more manageable and successful. Whether it's meal prep assistance, workout guidance, childcare support, or help with household chores, enlisting the help of others allows you to navigate logistical challenges with greater ease and focus more fully on your health and well-being. By leveraging the resources and expertise of your support network, you can overcome obstacles, stay motivated, and achieve lasting success in your weight loss goals.

4. Motivation and Inspiration

A support system serves as a reservoir of motivation and inspiration, fueling your determination and belief in your ability to achieve your weight loss goals. Within this network, you find role models, success stories, and a chorus of encouragement that propels you forward, even in the face of obstacles or setbacks.

One of the most significant sources of motivation within a support system is witnessing the success of others who have embarked on similar weight loss journeys. Whether it's a friend, family member, or member of an online community, seeing individuals who have achieved their goals can ignite a fire within you. Their triumphs serve as tangible evidence that success is possible, even in the face of challenges. By witnessing their transformation and hearing their stories of perseverance, you're reminded that your goals are within reach, motivating you to press on with renewed determination.

Moreover, a support system provides a platform for sharing experiences and insights, fostering a sense of camaraderie and solidarity among members. When you're surrounded by like-minded individuals who share your struggles and aspirations, you feel a sense of belonging and community that bolsters your confidence and determination. Whether it's swapping tips for overcoming cravings, celebrating milestones together, or offering words of encouragement during difficult times, the support and camaraderie of your peers can provide the strength and motivation needed to stay the course.

Additionally, within a support system, you may find mentors or role models who inspire you with their dedication, discipline, and achievements. These individuals serve as beacons of inspiration, demonstrating what's possible with perseverance and commitment. Whether it's a friend who consistently makes healthy choices or a fitness guru whose transformation story inspires awe, having role models to look up to can fuel your own determination to succeed. Their example reminds you that success is not just a distant dream but a tangible reality within your grasp, motivating you to stay committed to your goals.

Furthermore, the encouragement and support of your peers within a support system can provide the boost needed to overcome obstacles and setbacks along the way. When you're feeling discouraged or facing challenges, knowing that you have a network of individuals cheering you on can make all the difference. Their words of encouragement, empathy, and support serve as a lifeline, reminding you that you're not alone in your journey and encouraging you to keep pushing forward.

In conclusion, a support system is a powerful source of motivation and inspiration in your weight loss journey. Whether it's witnessing the success of others, sharing experiences and insights with like-minded individuals, or drawing inspiration from mentors and role models, the support of your peers can fuel your determination and belief in what's possible. By surrounding yourself with positive influences and tapping into the strength of your support network, you can stay motivated, overcome obstacles, and achieve lasting success in your weight loss goals.

5. Celebrating Successes Together

The journey towards weight loss is not just about overcoming challenges; it's also about celebrating victories, big and small. Within a support system, you have the opportunity to share these triumphs with others, amplifying the joy and satisfaction of your accomplishments.

One of the most significant benefits of celebrating successes within a support system is the reinforcement of your progress. Whether it's reaching a milestone weight loss goal, completing a challenging workout, or making healthier choices in your daily life, acknowledging and celebrating these achievements reinforces your commitment to your goals. By recognizing how far you've come and the progress you've made, you're motivated to continue pushing forward and striving for even greater success.

Moreover, celebrating successes together strengthens your connections with others within your support system. Sharing your victories with friends, family members, or peers creates bonds of camaraderie and solidarity that deepen your relationships. When you celebrate each other's successes, you foster a sense of mutual support and encouragement that strengthens the fabric of your support network. These shared experiences create lasting memories and strengthen the bonds of friendship, providing a source of strength and support as you continue your journey towards better health.

Furthermore, celebrating successes within a support system provides a sense of camaraderie and shared purpose that enhances your overall well-being. When you share your achievements with others who understand the challenges you've faced and the effort you've put in, you feel a sense of validation and recognition that boosts your self-esteem and confidence. Additionally, celebrating together creates a positive and uplifting atmosphere that fosters optimism, resilience, and a belief in what's possible. As you revel in each other's successes, you're inspired to continue pushing forward and striving for your own goals, knowing that you have a team of supporters cheering you on every step of the way.

In conclusion, celebrating successes together within a support system is an essential aspect of the weight loss journey. Whether it's recognizing milestones, accomplishments, or small victories along the way, sharing these moments with others amplifies the joy and satisfaction of your achievements. By reinforcing your progress, strengthening your connections with others, and fostering a sense of camaraderie and shared purpose, celebrating successes within a support system enhances your overall well-being and motivates you to continue pursuing your goals with determination and optimism.

Having a support system in your weight loss journey can significantly enhance your chances of success by providing emotional support, accountability, practical assistance, motivation, and opportunities for celebration. Whether it's friends, family members, workout buddies, or online communities, surrounding yourself with people who believe in you and support your goals can make all the difference in achieving lasting change. Cultivate and nurture your support system, lean on others when needed, and be open to offering support in return. Together, you can overcome obstacles, celebrate victories, and create a healthier, happier life.

CHAPTER 10: OVERCOMING PLATEAUS AND SETBACKS

The weight loss journey is often fraught with challenges that can test your resolve and determination. Among the most common hurdles are plateaus and setbacks, which can be discouraging and frustrating. However, understanding these challenges and learning how to navigate them can help you stay on track and achieve your weight loss goals. This chapter will delve into the nature of plateaus and setbacks, explore their causes, and offer strategies for overcoming them.

Understanding Plateaus

A weight loss plateau occurs when you stop losing weight despite maintaining your diet and exercise regimen. This stagnation can happen to anyone and is a normal part of the weight loss process. When you initially start losing weight, the changes in your lifestyle can lead to rapid weight loss. However, as your body adapts to these changes, the rate of weight loss can slow down and eventually stall.

Causes of Plateaus:

1. **Metabolic Adaptation**: As you lose weight, your body requires fewer calories to maintain its new weight. This is because a smaller body burns fewer calories at rest and during activity. Over time, your metabolism slows down, and the caloric deficit you created initially may no longer be sufficient for continued weight loss.

2. **Loss of Lean Muscle Mass**: Lean muscle mass burns more calories than fat. If you lose muscle along with fat, your metabolic rate decreases, contributing to a plateau.

3. **Consistency in Routine**: The body adapts to the same exercise routine over time. If your workouts become too predictable, they may no longer challenge your body, leading to a plateau.

Overcoming Plateaus:

1. **Reevaluate Your Caloric Intake**: As your weight decreases, so does your caloric requirement. Recalculate your daily caloric needs based on your current weight and adjust your intake accordingly.

2. **Increase Physical Activity**: Incorporate more physical activity into your routine. This can be achieved by increasing the intensity, duration, or frequency of your workouts. Adding variety to your exercise regimen, such as incorporating strength training, high-intensity interval training (HIIT), or new forms of cardio, can also help.

3. **Build Muscle**: Engage in strength training exercises to build lean muscle mass. This not only helps boost your metabolism but also improves your overall body composition.

4. **Monitor Macronutrient Ratios**: Sometimes, tweaking the balance of macronutrients (carbohydrates, proteins, and fats) in your diet can kickstart weight loss. Consult with a nutritionist to find the right balance for you.

5. **Stay Hydrated**: Drinking enough water is crucial for metabolism and can help you feel full, preventing overeating.

Understanding Setbacks

Setbacks are another common challenge in the weight loss journey. These can come in the form of weight regain, missed workouts, or lapses in healthy eating habits. Setbacks are often accompanied by feelings of guilt, frustration, and self-doubt, which can derail your progress if not managed effectively.

Causes of Setbacks:

1. **Emotional and Stress Eating**: Stress, anxiety, and emotional distress can trigger overeating or unhealthy food choices as a coping mechanism.

2. **Lack of Motivation**: Maintaining motivation over the long term can be difficult. Life events, holidays, or a busy schedule can cause you to lose focus on your weight loss goals.

3. **Unrealistic Expectations**: Setting overly ambitious goals can lead to disappointment and discouragement when they are not met, making it easier to give up.

4. **Social and Environmental Influences**: Social gatherings, peer pressure, and the availability of unhealthy food options can lead to lapses in healthy eating habits.

Overcoming Setbacks:

1. **Practice Self-Compassion**: Be kind to yourself and recognize that setbacks are a normal part of any journey. Avoid negative self-talk and focus on what you can learn from the experience.

2. **Identify Triggers**: Pay attention to the circumstances that lead to setbacks. Understanding your triggers can help you develop strategies to avoid or manage them in the future.

3. **Set Realistic Goals**: Break your weight loss goals into smaller, achievable milestones. Celebrate your successes along the way to stay motivated.

4. **Plan and Prepare**: Plan your meals and workouts in advance to avoid making impulsive decisions. Keep healthy snacks on hand to prevent overeating when you're hungry.

5. **Seek Support**: Lean on your support system for encouragement and accountability. Join a weight loss group or find a workout buddy to keep you motivated.

6. **Reframe Setbacks as Learning Opportunities**: Instead of viewing setbacks as failures, see them as opportunities to learn and grow. Analyze what went wrong and how you can prevent it from happening again.

7. **Get Back on Track Quickly**: Don't let a setback turn into a prolonged lapse. The sooner you resume your healthy habits, the less impact the setback will have on your overall progress.

8. **Practice Mindful Eating**: Be mindful of what and how much you eat. Pay attention to your hunger and fullness cues, and try to eat without distractions.

The Role of Professional Guidance

If you find yourself struggling with plateaus or setbacks despite your best efforts, seeking professional guidance can be beneficial. Dietitians, personal trainers, and mental health professionals can provide personalized advice and support tailored to your unique needs and challenges.

1. **Dietitians**: A registered dietitian can help you create a balanced and sustainable eating plan, ensuring you get the nutrients you need while maintaining a caloric deficit.

2. **Personal Trainers**: A personal trainer can design a customized workout plan that challenges your body and helps you build muscle, boosting your metabolism.

3. **Mental Health Professionals**: Addressing the emotional and psychological aspects of weight loss is crucial. Therapists or counselors can help you develop coping strategies for stress, emotional eating, and other mental obstacles.

Plateaus and setbacks are inevitable parts of the weight loss journey. They can be challenging, but they also offer opportunities for growth and self-improvement. By understanding the causes of these challenges and implementing strategies to overcome them, you can maintain your progress and achieve your weight loss goals. Remember, the journey is not just about reaching a destination but also about learning, adapting, and becoming stronger along the way. Stay committed, be patient with yourself, and celebrate every step forward, no matter how small.

CHAPTER 11: CELEBRATING PROGRESS

Embarking on a weight loss journey is a significant commitment that involves changing habits, overcoming challenges, and making continuous efforts to improve your health and well-being. While it's natural to focus on the ultimate goal, it's equally important to recognize and celebrate every success along the way, no matter how small. Acknowledging these milestones can provide motivation, reinforce positive behavior, and enhance your overall sense of accomplishment.

The Power of Positive Reinforcement
Positive reinforcement is a psychological principle that encourages the repetition of desired behaviors by rewarding them. When you celebrate small successes in your weight loss journey, you create a positive feedback loop that reinforces healthy habits and boosts your motivation. This principle can be applied in various ways:

1. **Setting Achievable Goals**: Break down your weight loss goal into smaller, manageable milestones. For instance, instead of focusing solely on losing 50 pounds, set intermediate goals such as losing 5 pounds, fitting into a specific piece of clothing, or consistently exercising three times a week. Each of these achievements is a step towards your ultimate goal and deserves recognition.

2. **Rewarding Yourself**: Treat yourself to non-food rewards when you reach a milestone. This could be anything from a new workout outfit, a relaxing spa day, or a fun outing with friends. These rewards provide tangible incentives that make the journey more enjoyable and satisfying.

Recognizing Non-Scale Victories

While the number on the scale is a common measure of weight loss success, it's not the only indicator of progress. Non-scale victories (NSVs) are equally important and can include a wide range of achievements related to health, fitness, and well-being:

1. **Improved Physical Fitness**: Celebrate improvements in your physical abilities, such as running a longer distance, lifting heavier weights, or completing a challenging workout. These accomplishments reflect your growing strength and endurance.

2. **Enhanced Health Metrics**: Pay attention to changes in your health metrics, such as lower blood pressure, improved cholesterol levels, or better blood sugar control. These improvements are direct results of your efforts and have a significant impact on your overall health.

3. **Positive Changes in Appearance**: Notice the changes in your body, such as increased muscle tone, a slimmer waistline, or glowing skin. These physical transformations are visible signs of your hard work and dedication.

4. **Increased Energy and Vitality**: Acknowledge the boost in your energy levels and overall sense of vitality. Feeling more energetic and capable of tackling daily tasks is a rewarding outcome of your healthier lifestyle.

5. **Improved Mental and Emotional Well-Being**: Recognize the positive impact of weight loss on your mental and emotional health. This might include reduced stress, improved mood, and a greater sense of confidence and self-esteem.

Creating a Habit of Celebration

To make celebrating your successes a regular part of your weight loss journey, consider incorporating the following practices:

1. **Keep a Success Journal**: Maintain a journal where you record your daily or weekly achievements, no matter how small. This could include sticking to your meal plan, completing a workout, or resisting a tempting treat. Reflecting on these successes can boost your morale and remind you of the progress you've made.

2. **Share Your Achievements**: Share your milestones with supportive friends, family members, or online communities. Celebrating with others can amplify your sense of accomplishment and provide additional encouragement.

3. **Create a Visual Progress Tracker**: Use a visual tool, such as a chart, graph, or progress photos, to track your journey. Seeing your progress in a tangible form can be incredibly motivating and help you stay focused on your goals.

Celebrating Through Self-Care

Self-care is an essential component of the weight loss journey and can serve as a meaningful way to celebrate your successes. By prioritizing self-care, you reinforce the idea that your health and well-being are worth the effort. Here are some self-care ideas to consider:

1. **Indulge in Relaxation**: Treat yourself to activities that promote relaxation and stress relief, such as a massage, a hot bath, or a quiet evening with a good book. These moments of relaxation can help recharge your body and mind.

2. **Engage in Enjoyable Activities**: Dedicate time to activities that bring you joy and fulfillment, whether it's a hobby, a creative pursuit, or spending time in nature.

Engaging in enjoyable activities can provide a mental break and remind you of the pleasures beyond the weight loss journey.

3. **Practice Mindfulness and Gratitude**: Incorporate mindfulness practices, such as meditation or deep breathing, into your daily routine. Additionally, cultivate a habit of gratitude by regularly acknowledging the positive aspects of your journey and expressing thanks for your progress and the support you receive.

Overcoming the Fear of Self-Congratulation

Some individuals may hesitate to celebrate their successes due to a fear of complacency or a belief that they don't deserve recognition until they reach their ultimate goal. It's important to challenge these notions and understand that celebrating small victories is not about settling for less but about acknowledging your efforts and sustaining motivation.

1. **Reframe Your Perspective**: View each small success as a building block towards your larger goal. Celebrating these achievements is a way to honor the hard work you've put in and to maintain momentum.

2. **Recognize Your Worth**: Understand that you are deserving of recognition and celebration at every stage of your journey. Your efforts and progress are valuable, regardless of how far you have left to go.

3. **Balance Celebration with Continued Effort**: Celebrating small successes doesn't mean you're finished; it's a way to reinforce positive behavior and stay motivated. Use these celebrations as fuel to continue striving towards your ultimate goals.

The Long-Term Benefits of Celebrating Successes

Celebrating your weight loss successes, no matter how small, has long-term benefits that extend beyond the immediate sense of accomplishment. These benefits include:

1. **Sustained Motivation**: Regularly acknowledging and celebrating your progress helps maintain high levels of motivation and commitment to your goals.

2. **Improved Self-Esteem**: Recognizing your achievements boosts your self-esteem and confidence, which can positively impact other areas of your life.

3. **Resilience in the Face of Challenges**: Celebrating successes builds resilience by reinforcing your ability to overcome obstacles and achieve your goals. This resilience can help you navigate future challenges with greater ease.

4. **Positive Reinforcement of Healthy Habits**: Celebrating your progress reinforces the healthy habits you've developed, making them more likely to become permanent parts of your lifestyle.

The journey to weight loss and improved health is a marathon, not a sprint. Along the way, it's essential to celebrate every step forward, no matter how small. By recognizing and honoring your successes, you create a positive feedback loop that sustains motivation, boosts self-esteem, and reinforces healthy behaviors. Remember, every achievement, no matter how minor it may seem, is a testament to your dedication and hard work. Celebrate them, cherish them, and let them propel you toward your ultimate goals.

Non-Food Rewards for Your Weight Loss Journey

Each step towards your weight loss goal deserves recognition and celebration. However, rewarding yourself with food can sometimes counteract your efforts and set back your progress.

Instead, consider non-food rewards that can provide motivation, satisfaction, and encouragement without compromising your health goals. This chapter will explore various non-food rewards you can use to celebrate your successes and keep your weight loss journey enjoyable and fulfilling.

The Importance of Non-Food Rewards

Non-food rewards are essential because they reinforce your progress and dedication in a way that aligns with your health goals. By choosing rewards that don't involve food, you avoid the risk of associating success with eating, which can lead to unhealthy patterns and emotional eating. Non-food rewards can help you:

1. **Reinforce Positive Behavior**: Celebrating achievements with non-food rewards encourages you to continue making healthy choices.

2. **Maintain Motivation**: Regularly rewarding yourself keeps you motivated and committed to your goals.

3. **Boost Self-Esteem**: Acknowledging your successes improves your self-esteem and confidence.

4. **Enjoy the Journey**: Rewards make the journey enjoyable, preventing burnout and frustration.

Ideas for Non-Food Rewards

Here are some creative and meaningful non-food rewards to consider as you celebrate your weight loss milestones:

1. **Fitness Gear and Accessories**:

   - **New Workout Clothes**: Treat yourself to a stylish workout outfit. New clothes can boost your confidence and make exercising more enjoyable.

- **Fitness Equipment**: Invest in home exercise equipment like resistance bands, a yoga mat, or dumbbells.

- **Fitness Tracker**: A fitness tracker can help you monitor your progress and stay motivated.

- **Sports Accessories**: Buy a new pair of running shoes, a swim cap, or cycling gear.

2. **Self-Care and Wellness**:

- **Massage or Spa Day**: Relax and rejuvenate with a professional massage or a spa day.

- **Manicure or Pedicure**: Pamper yourself with a manicure or pedicure.

- **Skincare Products**: Invest in high-quality skincare products or enjoy a facial treatment.

- **Aromatherapy**: Purchase essential oils or aromatherapy diffusers to create a calming environment at home.

3. **Hobbies and Personal Interests**:

- **Books and Magazines**: Buy a new book or subscribe to a magazine that interests you.

- **Craft Supplies**: Invest in supplies for a hobby, such as painting, knitting, or scrapbooking.

- **Music and Instruments**: Purchase new music or an instrument if you enjoy playing.

- **Gardening Tools**: Buy plants or tools for gardening if you have a green thumb.

4. **Experiences and Activities**:

   - **Concert or Event Tickets**: Treat yourself to a concert, theater show, or sports event.

   - **Classes and Workshops**: Enroll in a class or workshop that interests you, such as cooking, dancing, or photography.

   - **Travel and Getaways**: Plan a day trip, weekend getaway, or longer vacation to explore new places.

   - **Outdoor Adventures**: Try activities like hiking, kayaking, or camping.

5. **Home and Lifestyle**:

   - **Home Decor**: Redecorate a room or buy a new piece of furniture or art for your home.

   - **Tech Gadgets**: Purchase a new gadget, such as a tablet, smartwatch, or headphones.

   - **Subscription Services**: Subscribe to a service like a streaming platform, audiobook membership, or fitness app.

   - **Organizational Tools**: Invest in organizers, planners, or storage solutions to simplify your life.

6. **Social and Supportive Rewards**:

  - **Time with Loved Ones**: Plan a special outing or activity with friends or family.

  - **Recognition and Praise**: Share your achievements with your support system and let them celebrate with you.

  - **Joining a Community**: Participate in a group or community related to your interests or fitness goals.

Implementing Non-Food Rewards

To effectively incorporate non-food rewards into your weight loss journey, consider the following strategies:

1. **Set Specific Goals**: Clearly define your milestones and the rewards you'll give yourself for reaching them. This could include weight loss goals, fitness achievements, or consistency in healthy habits.

2. **Create a Reward System**: Develop a system where you earn points or tokens for your accomplishments. Once you accumulate enough points, you can redeem them for a reward.

3. **Be Consistent**: Regularly reward yourself for both small and significant achievements. Consistent rewards reinforce positive behavior and maintain motivation.

4. **Personalize Your Rewards**: Choose rewards that are meaningful and enjoyable to you. Personalization ensures that the rewards truly motivate and satisfy you.

5. **Celebrate with Others**: Involve friends and family in your celebrations. Their encouragement and recognition can amplify your sense of accomplishment.

The Long-Term Benefits of Non-Food Rewards

Using non-food rewards to celebrate your weight loss journey offers several long-term benefits:

1. **Sustainable Motivation**: Non-food rewards provide ongoing motivation, helping you stay committed to your goals over the long term.

2. **Healthier Relationships with Food**: By separating rewards from food, you develop a healthier relationship with eating and avoid using food as a source of comfort or reward.

3. **Enhanced Well-Being**: Non-food rewards often promote overall well-being, whether through physical activity, relaxation, or personal growth.

4. **Continued Personal Development**: Many non-food rewards, such as classes, hobbies, and experiences, contribute to your personal development and enrich your life beyond your weight loss journey.

In conclusion, celebrating your weight loss successes with non-food rewards is a powerful strategy that reinforces your commitment, boosts motivation, and enhances your overall well-being. By choosing rewards that align with your health goals and personal interests, you create a positive feedback loop that makes the journey enjoyable and fulfilling. Remember, every achievement, no matter how small, deserves recognition and celebration. Embrace the joy of rewarding yourself in meaningful ways, and let these celebrations propel you toward your ultimate goals.

CHAPTER 12: MAINTAINING WEIGHT LOSS

Achieving weight loss is a significant accomplishment, but maintaining that loss over the long term can be even more challenging. Sustained weight management requires ongoing commitment and lifestyle adjustments. This chapter will discuss effective strategies to help you maintain your weight loss and continue living a healthy, balanced life.

Understand Your Motivation

The first step in maintaining weight loss is to understand and continually revisit your motivation for losing weight in the first place. Reflect on the reasons that drove you to embark on your weight loss journey, such as improving your health, increasing energy levels, or boosting self-confidence. Keeping these motivations at the forefront of your mind can help you stay focused and committed to maintaining your new weight.

Develop a Sustainable Eating Plan

A sustainable eating plan is crucial for long-term weight maintenance. This plan should include a balanced diet that provides all the necessary nutrients without excessive calories. Here are some key components of a sustainable eating plan:

- **Balanced Diet**: Ensure your diet includes a variety of foods from all food groups, including fruits, vegetables, lean proteins, whole grains, and healthy fats. This variety provides essential nutrients and helps prevent boredom with your meals.

- **Portion Control**: Continue to practice portion control to avoid overeating. Use smaller plates and be mindful of serving sizes, especially when eating out or consuming packaged foods.

- **Mindful Eating**: Practice mindful eating by paying attention to your hunger and fullness cues. Eat slowly, savor each bite, and avoid distractions like watching TV or using electronic devices while eating.

- **Occasional Treats**: Allow yourself occasional treats to avoid feeling deprived. Moderation is key, so enjoy your favorite foods in small amounts without guilt.

Regular Physical Activity

Physical activity plays a vital role in maintaining weight loss. Regular exercise helps burn calories, build and maintain muscle mass, and boost your metabolism. Incorporate a mix of aerobic and strength-training exercises into your routine:

- **Aerobic Exercise**: Engage in at least 150 minutes of moderate-intensity aerobic exercise or 75 minutes of vigorous-intensity exercise per week. Activities like walking, jogging, cycling, and swimming are excellent options.

- **Strength Training**: Include strength training exercises at least twice a week to build and maintain muscle mass. This can include weightlifting, resistance band exercises, or bodyweight exercises like push-ups and squats.

- **Active Lifestyle**: Look for opportunities to stay active throughout the day, such as taking the stairs, walking or biking instead of driving, and incorporating short activity breaks into your daily routine.

Monitor Your Progress

Regularly monitoring your progress can help you stay on track with your weight maintenance goals. Here are some effective ways to monitor your progress:

- **Weigh Yourself**: Weigh yourself regularly, but not obsessively. Weekly weigh-ins can help you stay aware of any weight fluctuations and allow you to make adjustments if needed.

- **Track Your Food Intake**: Keep a food journal or use a mobile app to track your food intake. This can help you stay mindful of your eating habits and identify any patterns that may lead to weight gain.

- **Monitor Physical Activity**: Use a fitness tracker or app to monitor your physical activity levels. Setting and achieving daily or weekly activity goals can keep you motivated and accountable.

Build a Support System

A strong support system is essential for long-term weight maintenance. Surround yourself with people who encourage and support your healthy lifestyle choices:

- **Friends and Family**: Share your goals with friends and family members who can provide encouragement and accountability.

- **Support Groups**: Join a weight maintenance or fitness support group, either in person or online. Sharing your experiences and challenges with others who are on a similar journey can provide motivation and camaraderie.

- **Professional Support**: Consider working with a registered dietitian, personal trainer, or health coach for personalized guidance and support.

Manage Stress and Emotional Eating

Stress and emotional eating can undermine your weight maintenance efforts. Develop strategies to manage stress and cope with emotions without turning to food:

- **Stress Management Techniques**: Practice stress management techniques such as deep breathing, meditation, yoga, or progressive muscle relaxation to reduce stress levels.

- **Healthy Coping Mechanisms**: Identify healthy ways to cope with emotions, such as talking to a friend, engaging in a hobby, or going for a walk.

- **Mindful Eating**: Continue to practice mindful eating to stay aware of emotional triggers that may lead to overeating.

Stay Flexible and Adapt

Life is full of changes and challenges, and your weight maintenance plan should be flexible enough to adapt to different situations. Here are some tips for staying flexible:

- **Plan for Special Occasions**: Develop strategies for handling special occasions and holidays, such as portion control, choosing healthier options, and allowing yourself to enjoy treats in moderation.

- **Adjust Your Routine**: Be willing to adjust your exercise and eating routines as needed to accommodate changes in your schedule, such as travel, work commitments, or family responsibilities.

- **Stay Positive**: Maintain a positive attitude and focus on progress rather than perfection. Accept that occasional setbacks are a normal part of the journey and use them as learning opportunities.

Focus on Long-Term Health

Shift your focus from short-term weight loss goals to long-term health and well-being. This mindset can help you maintain healthy habits for life:

- **Set New Goals**: Continuously set new health and fitness goals to stay motivated and challenged. These goals could include improving your fitness level, trying new activities, or achieving specific health markers like lower blood pressure or cholesterol levels.

- **Celebrate Non-Scale Victories**: Recognize and celebrate non-scale victories, such as increased energy levels, improved mood, better sleep, and enhanced physical fitness.

- **Educate Yourself**: Stay informed about nutrition, fitness, and wellness to make knowledgeable choices and adapt to new information.

Maintaining weight loss in the long term requires ongoing commitment, flexibility, and a focus on overall health and well-being. By developing sustainable eating habits, staying physically active, monitoring your progress, building a support system, managing stress, and staying adaptable, you can successfully maintain your weight loss and enjoy a healthier, more fulfilling life. Remember that weight maintenance is a lifelong journey, and celebrating your progress and achievements along the way is essential to staying motivated and positive.

Preventing relapse is also a crucial aspect of maintaining weight loss and ensuring long-term success in your health and fitness journey. After achieving weight loss goals, it's common to face challenges that can lead to regaining lost weight. This chapter provides practical tips to help you prevent relapse and stay on track with your weight maintenance goals.

Understand and Accept the Possibility of Relapse

The first step in preventing relapse is to understand and accept that it can happen. Weight maintenance is a lifelong journey, and there may be times when you face setbacks. Recognizing this possibility allows you to prepare mentally and emotionally for such occurrences, reducing the likelihood of becoming discouraged or giving up altogether.

Stay Vigilant and Self-Aware

Staying vigilant and self-aware of your habits and behaviors is essential in preventing relapse. Here are some strategies to help you stay mindful:

- **Regular Self-Monitoring**: Continue to monitor your weight, food intake, and physical activity levels regularly. Keeping track of these factors helps you stay aware of any changes that could lead to weight gain.

- **Reflect on Triggers**: Identify and reflect on triggers that may lead to overeating or unhealthy habits. These could include stress, emotional distress, social situations, or specific foods. Understanding your triggers allows you to develop strategies to manage them effectively.

- **Mindful Eating**: Practice mindful eating by paying attention to your hunger and fullness cues. Eat slowly, savor each bite, and avoid distractions such as watching TV or using electronic devices while eating.

Maintain a Balanced Diet

A balanced diet is fundamental in preventing relapse. Here are some tips to help you maintain healthy eating habits:

- **Nutrient-Dense Foods**: Focus on consuming nutrient-dense foods such as fruits, vegetables, lean proteins, whole grains, and healthy fats. These foods provide essential nutrients while keeping you satisfied.

- **Portion Control**: Continue to practice portion control to avoid overeating. Use smaller plates and bowls, and be mindful of serving sizes, especially when dining out or eating packaged foods.

- **Regular Meals**: Stick to regular meal times and avoid skipping meals, which can lead to overeating later in the day. Balanced meals and snacks help maintain energy levels and prevent excessive hunger.

Incorporate Regular Physical Activity

Regular physical activity is crucial for preventing relapse and maintaining weight loss. Here are some tips to help you stay active:

- **Variety in Exercise**: Incorporate a variety of exercises into your routine to keep things interesting and prevent boredom. Include aerobic activities, strength training, and flexibility exercises.

- **Active Lifestyle**: Look for opportunities to stay active throughout the day, such as taking the stairs, walking or biking instead of driving, and incorporating short activity breaks into your daily routine.

Seek Professional Help if Needed

If you find yourself struggling to maintain your weight loss or facing persistent challenges, consider seeking professional help. A registered dietitian, therapist, or counselor can provide additional support and guidance to help you overcome obstacles and stay on track.

Preventing relapse in your weight loss journey requires ongoing commitment, self-awareness, and adaptability. By staying vigilant, maintaining a balanced diet, incorporating regular physical activity, building a strong support system, managing stress, and focusing on long-term health, you can successfully maintain your weight loss and continue living a healthy, balanced life. Remember that setbacks are a natural part of the journey, and practicing self-compassion and seeking support when needed can help you overcome challenges and stay motivated.

CHAPTER 13: CONCLUSION AND NEXT STEPS

As we reach the conclusion of this book, it's essential to reflect on the key takeaways and the valuable lessons that can support you on your journey towards a healthier lifestyle. Achieving and maintaining weight loss is a multifaceted process that involves understanding nutrition, incorporating physical activity, managing stress, and building a strong support system. Let's summarize the critical points covered and provide encouragement to keep you motivated and inspired.

Understanding Nutrition and Its Role in Weight Loss
One of the foundational elements of successful weight loss is understanding the principles of nutrition:

1. **Balanced Diet**: A balanced diet rich in fruits, vegetables, lean proteins, whole grains, and healthy fats is crucial. It provides the necessary nutrients for overall health while supporting weight loss.

2. **Portion Control**: Managing portion sizes helps regulate calorie intake. Using smaller plates, being mindful of serving sizes, and avoiding oversized portions, especially when eating out, can prevent overeating.

3. **Hydration**: Drinking adequate water promotes feelings of fullness and prevents dehydration, which can sometimes be mistaken for hunger.

4. **Mindful Eating**: Paying attention to hunger and fullness cues, eating slowly, and savoring each bite helps avoid mindless eating and overeating.

The Importance of Physical Activity

Physical activity plays a vital role in weight loss and overall health:

1. **Regular Exercise**: Incorporating regular physical activity, including both aerobic exercises and strength training, helps burn calories, build lean muscle mass, and improve overall fitness.

2. **Consistency**: Aim for at least 150 minutes of moderate-intensity aerobic exercise or 75 minutes of vigorous-intensity exercise per week, along with muscle-strengthening activities on two or more days per week.

3. **Enjoyable Activities**: Finding activities you enjoy makes it easier to stay motivated and consistent. This could be anything from walking and jogging to dancing, cycling, or swimming.

Building a Strong Support System

A robust support system is essential for maintaining motivation and accountability:

1. **Emotional Support**: Having friends, family, or online communities who understand and empathize with your struggles can provide comfort and encouragement during challenging times.

2. **Accountability Partners**: Workout buddies or friends who regularly check in on your progress can help you stay focused and committed to your goals.

3. **Professional Guidance**: Registered dietitians, personal trainers, or health coaches can provide personalized advice and support to help you achieve your goals.

Managing Stress and Emotional Eating

Stress and emotional eating are significant barriers to weight loss:

1. **Stress Management**: Techniques such as deep breathing, meditation, yoga, and progressive muscle relaxation can help reduce stress levels.

2. **Healthy Coping Mechanisms**: Identifying healthy ways to cope with emotions, such as talking to a friend, engaging in hobbies, or spending time in nature, can reduce reliance on food for comfort.

3. **Mindful Eating**: Practicing mindful eating helps you stay aware of emotional triggers and avoid using food to cope with stress.

The Role of Sleep in Weight Loss

Quality sleep is crucial for weight loss and overall health:

1. **Consistent Sleep Schedule**: Going to bed and waking up at the same time each day helps regulate your body's internal clock and promotes better sleep quality.

2. **Bedtime Routine**: Developing a calming bedtime routine, such as reading, taking a warm bath, or practicing relaxation techniques, signals to your body that it's time to wind down.

3. **Sleep Environment**: Keeping your bedroom cool, dark, and quiet, and minimizing distractions can improve sleep quality.

Preventing Relapse and Maintaining Weight Loss

Preventing relapse and maintaining weight loss requires ongoing effort and adaptation:

1. **Self-Monitoring**: Regularly monitoring your weight, food intake, and physical activity levels helps you stay aware of any changes that could lead to weight gain.

2. **Flexibility**: Being willing to adjust your exercise and eating routines to accommodate changes in your schedule can help you stay on track.

3. **Positive Mindset**: Maintaining a positive attitude and focusing on progress rather than perfection can help you stay motivated and resilient.

Celebrating Successes

Recognizing and celebrating your successes, no matter how small, is crucial for maintaining motivation:

1. **Non-Food Rewards**: Rewarding yourself with non-food items, such as new workout gear, a spa day, or a fun activity, can reinforce positive behavior and keep you motivated.

2. **Acknowledging Progress**: Celebrating milestones, such as reaching a weight loss goal, completing a challenging workout, or adopting healthier habits, helps reinforce your progress and boosts your confidence.

As you move forward, it's essential to remember that weight loss and maintaining a healthy lifestyle is a lifelong journey. Here are some final pieces of encouragement to keep you motivated and inspired:

Stay Committed to Your Goals

Commitment is key to long-term success. Remind yourself of your reasons for wanting to lose weight and maintain a healthy lifestyle. Whether it's to improve your health, boost your confidence, or increase your energy levels, keeping your goals in mind can help you stay focused and motivated.

Be Patient and Kind to Yourself

Weight loss is not a linear process, and setbacks are a natural part of the journey. Be patient with yourself and recognize that progress takes time. Practice self-compassion and treat yourself with kindness, especially during challenging times. Remember that every small step you take brings you closer to your goals.

Continue Learning and Growing

Stay informed about nutrition, fitness, and wellness to make knowledgeable choices and adapt to new information. Continuously setting new health and fitness goals can keep you motivated and challenged. Embrace the journey as an opportunity to learn and grow, both physically and mentally.

Surround Yourself with Positive Influences

Surrounding yourself with positive influences can significantly impact your motivation and success. Seek out friends, family members, or communities that support and encourage your healthy lifestyle choices. Sharing your experiences and challenges with others who are on a similar journey can provide motivation and camaraderie.

Celebrate Your Successes

Recognize and celebrate your successes, no matter how small. Celebrating your achievements reinforces your progress and provides a sense of accomplishment. Take pride in your hard work and dedication, and use your successes as motivation to keep pushing forward.

Seek Professional Support if Needed

If you find yourself struggling or facing persistent challenges, don't hesitate to seek professional support. A registered dietitian, therapist, or counselor can provide additional guidance and support to help you overcome obstacles and stay on track.

Embarking on a weight loss journey is a courageous and transformative decision. By understanding the principles of nutrition, incorporating regular physical activity, building a strong support system, managing stress, prioritizing sleep, and maintaining a positive mindset, you can achieve and maintain your weight loss goals. Remember that this journey is unique to you, and it's important to find what works best for your lifestyle and preferences.

Stay committed, be patient, and continue to celebrate your progress along the way. With determination, resilience, and support, you can create a healthier, happier, and more fulfilling life. Here's to your ongoing success and well-being!

ABOUT THE AUTHOR

Evelyn Inkwell, a renowned fitness expert in her 30s, has dedicated her career to the fields of weight management and fitness. With many years of hands-on experience, Evelyn has become a trusted authority in helping individuals achieve their fitness goals in a healthy and sustainable manner. Her journey in the fitness world began with a deep passion for health and wellness, which she now channels into her writing to inspire and guide others.

Evelyn's extensive background in fitness and weight management is reflected in her practical and empathetic approach to wellness. She understands the challenges that come with striving for a healthier lifestyle and offers valuable insights that are rooted in real-world experience. Her books are a testament to her commitment to providing readers with the knowledge and tools they need to succeed.

Driven by a mission to help everyone live a healthy life, Evelyn Inkwell writes with a genuine desire to make a positive impact on her readers' lives. Her work is characterized by its accessibility, motivational tone, and evidence-based strategies, making her a beloved figure among those seeking to transform their health and fitness. Evelyn's dedication to her craft and her unwavering support for her readers' journeys make her a standout author in the field of weight loss and management.